# The Essential Guide to Public Health and Health Promotion

In the twenty-first century, public health is everyone's business. The nursing and medical professions are well placed to provide advice to their clients, especially in respect to lifestyle change, and public health initiatives are supported by a range of statutory and voluntary organisations and health workers, ranging from health promotion specialists to smoking cessation advisers and nutrition assistants.

Designed to help readers develop the practical skills they need to become effective public health practitioners, this concise text gives an easily digested overview of public health and health promotion theory in accessible language and diagrams, before moving on to the ways readers can apply this in practice.

Providing an opportunity for practitioners to understand possible barriers to lifestyle change, debate health inequalities and responsibilities, and explore the role of the media in changing attitudes, this book:

- outlines the roles of specific organisations involved in public health work;
- covers health needs assessment, agenda setting and the technical aspects of how to research, plan and evaluate effective practice either with individual clients or when devising programmes and initiatives for population groups;
- details methods of helping people with motivation for lifestyle change, building rapport, ongoing support, monitoring and signposting to specific services;
- discusses the role of neighbourhoods and communities in improving health and how workers may support local populations to improve the health of their community.

*The Essential Guide to Public Health and Health Promotion* is an accessible introduction to the principles and practice of health promotion and public health for all those new to working or studying in the area, whatever their professional background.

**Susan R. Thompson** has worked in the field of public health for over twenty-five years within nursing, health promotion and academia. She currently holds the post of Course Lead for Graduate Entry Nursing at the University of Nottingham, UK, and has published a range of articles and delivered international conference presentations and workshops on public health.

# The Essential Guide to Public Health and Health Promotion

Susan R. Thompson

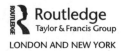

Routledge
Taylor & Francis Group

LONDON AND NEW YORK

First published 2014
by Routledge
2 Park Square, Milton Park, Abingdon, Oxon, OX14 4RN

and by Routledge
711 Third Avenue, New York, NY 10017

*Routledge is an imprint of the Taylor & Francis Group, an informa business*

*British Library Cataloguing in Publication Data*
A catalogue record for this book is available from the British Library

*Library of Congress Cataloging-in-Publication Data*
  Thompson, Susan R. (Susan Rosemary), 1961– author.
  The essential guide to public health and health promotion /
  Susan R. Thompson.
  p. ; cm.
  Includes bibliographical references.
  I. Title.
  [DNLM: 1. Public Health Practice.  2. Health Promotion. WA 100]
  RA425
  362.1—dc23
  2013040153

ISBN: 978–0–415–81307–5 (hbk)
ISBN: 978–0–415–81308–2 (pbk)
ISBN: 978–0–203–06832–8 (ebk)

Typeset in Sabon by
Swales & Willis Ltd, Exeter, Devon, UK

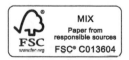

Printed and bound by CPI Group (UK) Ltd, Croydon, CR0 4YY

# Contents

# Illustrations

## Figures

## Tables

## Boxes

# Contributors

**Mo Almond** is a member of the Motivational Interviewing Network of Trainers and has had over thirty years' experience of working with people of all ages and backgrounds across a broad spectrum of health-related settings. The majority of her career has been spent in the field of public health and specialist health promotion, working to reduce health inequalities and improve health outcomes on a population and individual basis. Following a person centred counselling course Mo became increasingly interested in the psychology of behaviour change, in particular motivational interviewing. In 2003 she attended the internationally recognised training the trainers course run by Drs William Miller and Stephen Rollnick (MINT) and has since been delivering MI training and coaching to a rich diversity of practitioners from the fields of health, well-being, education and social care.

**Vicky Baldwin** is an education practice consultant with the UK Institute of Mental Health. She is also the lead for the BSc Knowledge and Understanding Framework. This is a national framework to support people to work more effectively with personality disorder, the main goal being to improve service user experience through developing the skills and knowledge of the multi-disciplinary workforce. Vicky has spoken at international conferences and published books and articles on mental health.

**Stephanie James** is a clinical nurse specialist and health promotion specialist (alcohol) for NHS Nottingham City. She holds a bachelor's degree in public health and primary care and a diploma in nursing. She is also an independent prescriber and holds a postgraduate certificate in alcohol and drug treatment. In 2009 Stephanie joined the charity Framework to help establish the Last Orders Alcohol Service, and has published in the *Journal of Community Nursing*.

**Vanessa McFarlane** has worked in the field of health promotion for over eighteen years. Her work has focused on sexual health, black and minority ethnic community health, child sexual exploitation and HIV. Vanessa has a bachelor's degree in social policy and administration from Nottingham University. She has successfully led a sexual health project targeting African and Caribbean communities, which has been in operation for ten years. She has coordinated the development and delivery of training, managed sexual health campaigns and written on BME men's health.

**Claire Novak** has worked as a health promotion specialist within Nottingham City for over twenty years, holding locality and public health commissioning roles. Currently she works in tobacco control. She received a BSc (Hons) in human ecology from the University of Huddersfield, and a postgraduate diploma, then an MSc in health promotion and health education from Leeds Metropolitan University, during which she conducted research into women and physical activity.

**Anne Pridgeon** is a registered dietician who gained a master's in public health in 2008. She has over twenty years of experience in public health and clinical dietetics, having worked in the areas of public health nutrition (including obesity), oral health, mental health and learning disabilities. She currently holds the post of Senior Public Health Manager at Nottinghamshire County Council and is responsible for the commissioning of programmes to prevent and treat obesity.

**Kate Thompson** is Tobacco Control Alliance Coordinator for Nottingham City Council. In this role she leads collective action to reduce smoking prevalence and builds on partnership working to ensure effective implementation of national tobacco control strategy at a local level. Her career to date has spanned three decades of working in the voluntary and public sectors, during which time she has gained a wide variety of experience across many areas including community development, self-help and health policy. Kate began working on the tobacco control agenda in 2005 and during that time she has been instrumental in developing a broad range of tobacco control interventions and awareness-raising campaigns. She is proud to be working to help achieve Nottingham City's vision of a smoke-free Nottingham.

**Susan R. Thompson** has worked in the field of public health for over twenty-five years within nursing, health promotion and academia. She currently holds the post of Course Lead for Graduate Entry Nursing at the University of Nottingham and leads on the adult field and problem-based learning aspect of the curriculum. She holds a master's in public health, is a fellow of the Higher Education Academy and acts as external examiner and advisor for two master's public health programmes. She has published a range of articles and delivered international conference presentations and workshops on public health. In 2012 she won the prestigious Lord Dearing Award for excellence in teaching and learning.

# Foreword

With the changes to the National Health Service, the initiation of health and well-being boards, the move of responsibility for the public's health to local authorities and the establishment of Public Health England, the need for clear thinking, coherence and practical advice on health promotion and education for public health practitioners has never been more important. However, as noted in Chapter 3, 'The NHS still has the monopoly for the medical approach to health promotion'. This book challenges this orthodoxy and offers practical applications for understanding the issues and avoiding simplistic solutions.

The importance of tackling the causes and results of disease, disability, disadvantage and health inequalities has never been greater as demand for health services, access to new treatments and specialist drugs increases at an ever faster rate, putting a strain on providers and services and a financial burden on both local and national resources. As ever, there are perceived 'winners and losers': individuals, families and communities, nationally and internationally. Chapter 2 draws attention to this issue and the dilemmas it raises, commenting that 'there are huge discrepancies in the standard of health individuals can expect throughout the world' dependent upon country, gender, age, ethnicity and income. Pointedly, as stated in Chapter 4:

> In England and Wales people who live in wealthier areas live on average up to fourteen years longer than those in poorer areas . . . Within society there is no doubt that judgements are made regarding prioritisation of needs; what might be seen as a need by one person may be seen as indulgent by another.

The Marmot Report argues that national and regional leadership should promote awareness of the underlying social causes of health inequalities and build understanding across the NHS, local government, third sector and private sector services of the need to scale up interventions and sustain intensity using mainstream funding. Interventions should have an evidence-based evaluation framework and a health equity impact assessment. This would help delivery organisations shape effective interventions, understand impacts of other policies on health distributions and avoid drift into small-scale projects focused on individual behaviour and lifestyle.

This book will help those engaged in health promotion and public health to approach health improvement, health protection and health care with confidence. It will help practitioners and those engaged in local government, the voluntary sector, the NHS and its partners to align their activities and provide improved outcomes for the public's health. It will help practitioners engage with the public and communities as well as helping to build workforce capacity. If we are to be successful, we need a workforce who are competent and confident as well as being passionate about improving health and well-being. Central to this is the need to use innovative approaches, especially evidence-based interventions underpinned by research.

In the early stages of reform Public Health England talked about transforming public health and creating a true 'wellness' service to meet today's public health challenge to improve health and protect against health hazards. In practice this will require practitioners to make use of data and evidence to inform practice and utilise social media and of course specialist expertise around the health and well-being priorities of tobacco, alcohol and substance misuse; nutrition, including diet, obesity and exercise; mental health; and sexual health, including HIV. Working with communities to plan interventions, as set out in Chapter 7, primary data

> gained from questionnaires, focus groups, social networks, voluntary organisations and neighbourhood groups are essential to achieve a picture of the perceived needs of the community in focus. This primary data married with the secondary epidemiological data and evidence gained from local authorities and health and social care services can create a complete picture of the community.

Finally, a cautionary note recognised in Chapter 1: 'Individuals rarely have complete control over their environment and the choices they make.' I believe it is essential for an individual's health that they are able to assess and evaluate information, manage risk and make lifestyle choices that develop, promote and maintain a healthy lifestyle and, ultimately, good health. This view of health literacy has to be more robust and empowering than those that simply require the passive ability to read, understand and act upon health information. This book goes a long way in helping practitioners in health promotion and public health to achieve this ambition.

Dr John Lloyd
President, Institute of Health Promotion and Education (IHPE)

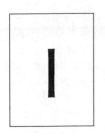

# What is health?

## Susan R. Thompson

Health is a term used widely in our society. People will state that they are in good health, and asking after one's health is one of the commonest forms of greeting. Yet we take little time to consider exactly what is meant by the term health. It is argued that health is in fact a social construct, that the meaning differs from society to society and from individual to individual depending on cultural values and norms and personal experiences and attitudes.

## Definitions of health

The World Health Organisation has defined health as 'a complete state of physical, mental and social well-being, and not merely the absence of disease or infirmity' (WHO 1986). This seems like a bit of a tall order, as it is doubtful that one individual can say that they exist in such a blessed state for any significant period of time, if at all. However, this definition was revolutionary at the time as it acknowledged that health should not be seen as purely a biological status and that psychological and social health was as important. A more nuanced definition is provided by Bircher (2005), who defines health as 'a dynamic state of well-being characterized by a physical and mental potential, which satisfies the demands of life commensurate with age, culture, and personal responsibility'. This takes account of how levels of good health will naturally vary with age and individual expectations.

### The biomedical model of health

Within Western societies the biomedical model of health prevails as the dominant model of health and until recently was largely unquestioned. Within this model, disease is seen as a defined state experienced by the body as a result of a pathological condition that is either temporary (curable) or permanent (incurable). The mind and body are seen as separate. The body is viewed as a functioning machine with all disease being explained by the physical working of the body, which, if disease is present, will need repairing. It is also a very interventionist model that is forever developing new techniques, tests and treatment to achieve a cure or alleviate symptoms (Nettleton 1995). Treatment on individuals is carried out by health professionals, primarily doctors, who perform tests, diagnose disease and prescribe treatment – either medication or surgery. The biomedical model of health has traditionally played up its curative success and downplayed the negative consequences or side effects of some of its treatments. Medical interventions can do harm as well as good. Overuse of antibiotic therapy, for example, has caused bacterial resistance, as was the case with the growth of Methicillin-resistant *Staphylococcus aureus* (MRSA). The biomedical model is familiar and is widely accepted and entrenched in our society. However, the model's complete dominance has been challenged in recent years as it has been tempered by influences from other cultures and a growing awareness of the role that society plays in health.

## *Other models of health*

Cultures around the world define health differently. Australian Aboriginal people generally define health as not just meaning the physical well-being of the individual but also the social, emotional, spiritual and cultural well-being of the whole community (NHMRC 1996). This is very different from the individualised Western way of viewing health. The Chinese see health as a balance of forces. For the body to remain healthy an equilibrium needs to be acquired between Yin (cold elements) and Yang (hot elements). Such a view is often the basis of alternative therapies and differs greatly from the Western biomedical approach to health. These alternative views are having an impact. Medical domination is lessening, people ask questions of their doctors and there is movement towards involving people in care, providing them with information so that the health care professionals and the patient can become partners in care. Until relatively recently there was a lack of acknowledgement of the part that lifestyle change could play in preventing ill health and still there is a lack of emphasis on the part that environment, social networks, income and employment, for example, can play in contributing towards health status. Gradually health and health care is being seen as achieving a balance between the body, the mind and the spirit and acknowledges the multiple factors that influence health.

## Influences on health

In order to become effective and efficient health promoters it is essential to broaden our minds away from the narrowness of the biomedical model and understand the complex interplay of factors affecting health. Some factors which influence our health are constitutional and cannot be altered – our genetics, our gender and our age are all such factors. However, many of the other influences we either impose on ourselves or are imposed upon us by the society in which we live. Some factors we have more control over than others; however, all factors are influenced by the way society is constructed. We may choose not to smoke tobacco, for instance, but this choice may be made harder for us if many of those within our social circle smoke. Some factors we have little choice over as individuals, for example whether we become a victim of crime, although there are actions we can take to lessen this risk. Table 1.1 gives a

Table 1.1 Health choices

| Choice | Dependent on | Controlled or influenced by |
|---|---|---|
| **Drinking alcohol** | Knowledge of safe alcohol limits<br>Availability of alcohol to individuals<br>Social acceptability amongst peers<br>Income to purchase<br>Access to drinking environment<br>Addiction services for those wanting to limit intake | Health educators<br>Licensing laws regarding premises, hours of sale, age limits for sale, responsible selling<br>Alcohol manufactures<br>Alcohol pricing<br>Number of purchasing outlets<br>Health policy and funding |
| **Cycling** | Income to purchase equipment<br>Individual ability to ride<br>Individual ability to store equipment<br>Individual motivation and enjoyment<br>Time available<br>Provision of safe environment | Cycling organisations, lobbying groups<br>Local authorities, transport and leisure departments, highways agency<br>Manufacturers of equipment<br>Cycle retailers<br>Workplace Cycle schemes |
| **Eating a healthy diet** | Knowledge of what constitutes a healthy diet<br>Individual and family motivation<br>Income to purchase healthy food<br>Cooking skills<br>Food storage, cooking and eating facilities | Health educators<br>Food standards agency<br>Farmers and food producers<br>Food manufacturers and retail agreements<br>Labelling guidelines<br>Food pricing |
| **Level of educational attainment** | Intellectual ability and motivation<br>Supportive family and cultural environment<br>Income to purchase equipment, e.g. computers, textbooks<br>Good quality educational environment<br>Good teachers<br>Cost of education to individual<br>Qualification infrastructure, exam boards, awarding bodies | Education acts – age and level of compulsory education by law<br>Level of Government and Local Authority funding for buildings and learning resources<br>Quality of teacher training<br>Educational watchdogs and quality control organisations |
| **Smoking cannabis** | Access to sales network for drug<br>Income to purchase<br>Social acceptability amongst peers<br>Addiction services for those wanting to quit<br>Education and prevention services | Drug laws<br>Police<br>Health educators<br>Health policy and funding |
| **Regular social contact** | Access to supportive social circle<br>Transport to meeting places<br>Individual motivation and skills<br>Income to purchase activities<br>Variety of activities available | Public and private transport infrastructure and funding<br>Regulation of safe activities<br>Groups of individuals with particular interests |

snapshot of some common influences on our health and illustrates the links between the choice the individual may choose to make, what that choice is dependent upon and what controls are exerted by society over that choice.

It can be seen from Table 1.1 that lifestyle choices are complex decisions, and it is important to see the bigger picture here as all too often individuals are held completely responsible for the way they live and the behaviour they exhibit. Unfortunately, individuals rarely have complete control over their environment and the choices they make. Any person who has found the motivation to make a positive behaviour change ought to be commended, as they are battling against the limitations that society places on them. That said, society also puts laws, guidelines, agreements and funding in place to aid positive behaviour change and to make healthy choices easier for individuals to make.

## Activity

Think about the following factors, and list the many ways each of these may negatively or positively affect health. Discussion of each of these factors is given at the end of this chapter.

Unemployment
The family we live with
The political system of the country
War
The standard of housing in which we live
Our level of self-confidence
Driving a car

## Perceptions of health

Sociologists have studied the ways various sectors of society perceive health and have proposed theories to explain these. Some people adhere to the functionalist model or way of looking at health. They ignore their health needs and tend to seek help only when a condition interferes with what they consider to be their optimal level of performance. They see themselves as healthy as long as they can perform their perceived roles and responsibilities in the workplace or in the home. Even if they are in pain or develop a rash or lose a certain degree of mobility, for example, as long as they can perform the necessary tasks in their daily lives they consider themselves to be healthy. This limited expectation of what constitutes health is a common one, especially amongst working class societies who generally have lower expectations of good health than do the affluent sectors of the population (Barry and Yull 2012). Different genders also view health differently. Men are much more likely to view their body as a machine that occasionally breaks down and needs to be fixed, and they are generally less likely to discuss symptoms with other men or seek help, often leaving problems until they have deteriorated to a dangerous degree. This attitude is a serious one, as from birth to the age of 75 years male mortality significantly outstrips that of female mortality (White and Cash 2003). It has been argued that this reluctance by men to access health care or indeed adopt preventative health measures is the result of the perceived need by men to conform to a masculine identity, one which values strength and decries weakness and ill health as a feminine indulgence (Arber and Cooper 2000). There are numerous examples of men waiting many months or years suspecting that various symptoms they are experiencing may be indicative of some disease but failing to present for investigation (ICR 2009). In 2009 research by Cancer Research UK found that men were 40 per cent more likely to die of cancer than women (Cohen 2009). Women tend to define health more in terms of social relationships than men, they tend to discuss symptoms more with each other and are more likely to present to health care professionals when they do have a problem (Barry and Yull 2012). Statistics show that between the ages of 5 and 75 men use health care services far less than women (ONS 2005). This may be the result of more emotional openness, but also women are generally brought into contact with health care services much more than the average man. Young women tend to seek contraceptive services, they may become pregnant and then later access health care with their children, and in middle age symptoms associated with the menopause may also make them seek help. This makes the average woman probably much more familiar with health care provision than the average man, who provided that he stays well may not access health care until late middle age. Given this circumstance it is not surprising that he is reluctant to enter a system about which he has no knowledge and, what is more, has to disclose intensely personal aspects of himself. Younger people are more likely to see health as an infinite resource. They value the physical fitness, strength and vitality they possess and cannot envisage ever being without this. This leads young people into more risk-taking behaviour than older groups. People in middle age have a more rounded notion of health that incorporates a feeling of mental and social well-being as well as physical functioning. Older people have lower expectations of good health, they generally expect to have aches and pains and have less physical prowess than when they were younger. However, they value their ability to live independent lives and perform common tasks and daily routines, and this becomes their benchmark for health. There seems to be a reluctance to be seen as being ill and a strong motivation towards feeling and being seen as healthy (Blaxter 2004). The obvious difficulty is that, as health means so many different things to different people, it is quite a task to be able to positively influence health, to promote good health.

## Perceptions of illness

The above raises the question that if there are differing opinions to what constitutes health it is logical that there is the same issue with what constitutes ill health. Often ill health is perceived by the individual as something that differs from the norm. In one South American tribe, a disfiguring skin condition has become so widespread within the population that it is considered the normal or healthy state. So distorted is this perception that the few individuals free of the infection are considered abhorrent and are refused the right to marry and pass on their immunity to succeeding generations

(Zola 1983). However, it isn't just in primitive societies that such situations occur; in Western societies ill health is also socially constructed to some extent. Societal accept- ability plays a role in defining ill health. In the Victorian era, women who transgressed societal norms and had affairs and illegitimate offspring ran the risk of being diagnosed insane and committed to asylums. In developed nations people who state that they can hear voices are likely to receive a diagnosis of schizophrenia and receive medication to block these. In primitive societies such a person may be revered as being able to speak to the spirit world and declared a highly respected Shaman. Attitudes to disability is an excellent example of how things have changed. Until recently, disabled children were placed in special schools and considered to have no future in contributing positively to society; rather they would need care for the rest of their lives, by the state and their families. During the last thirty years or so attitudes have changed; disability labels have altered from 'retarded' to 'mentally handicapped', through 'differently abled' to 'special needs', and this might not be the end of it. The aim is to present a positive view of dis- ability, a social model rather than a medical model. In the social model the emphasis is on how society needs to change in order for the disabled to be integrated into and contribute to society, whereas the medical model focused on the problems the disabled person had and how to change or fix them in order that they fitted into society as it is (ODI 2012). The result has largely been a sea change in attitudes to disability; the disa- bled have commanded much more respect and greater expectations are placed on them. The 2012 London Paralympic Games did much to increase respect for disabled athletes. However, adjectives such as 'superhuman' did the Paralympians and the disabled little service, with disability charities voicing concern in the press that this may raise questions about the need for disablement benefits (*The Independent* 2012). It seems that society has to swing from one extreme to the other before it reaches the middle ground.

## What is public health?

### Definitions of public health

The most well-recognised definition of public health is perhaps the following: 'The sci- ence and art of preventing disease, prolonging life and promoting health through the organised efforts and informed choices of society, organisations, public and private, communities and individuals' (Winslow 1920 cited by Viseltear 1982). Although writ- ten in the 1920s, the definition stands the test of time. Public health is about reducing mortality rates, but also about improving quality of life. This definition also introduces the idea that promoting health is everyone's responsibility. Individuals make choices that affect health, but also, as we have seen, the way society acts and is constructed affects health. National and local government play a part within this, as do health services, employers, community groups, families and so on – the list goes on and on. Winslow also acknowledges with the phrase 'science and art' that it is not solely medi- cal discoveries that contribute to good health – important though these are – but also the less defined factors that contribute to the way we feel. Our social relationships, the environment we live in and our sense of purpose may be some of the factors he consid- ered to be the arts of public health.

## The work of public health

Perhaps it is also useful to discuss the principles of public health practice. Healthworks (2001), a forum that styles itself as being made up of the world's best thinkers in health care, has stated the following principles as being essential to public health:

- To improve the health and well-being of populations, communities, families and individuals.
- To prevent disease and minimise its consequences.
- To prolong valued life.
- To reduce inequalities in health.

These are in general agreement with Winslow; the only difference is the inclusion of the principle to reduce inequalities in health. This has become a fundamental goal in public health in recent decades and will be discussed in more depth in the following chapter. Added to this should be health surveillance. This work is the collection of data about the prevalence and incidence of disease and lifestyle factors that lead to disease. Statistics in the UK are generally collated by the Office for National Statistics and the Public Health Observatories, but health professionals, charities, public bodies and researchers all contribute to this essential gathering of information, without which it would be impossible to know the extent of problems, the trend of those problems and indeed if interventions are proving to be effective.

## Health promotion

Health promotion is an important arm of public health practice and has been defined as 'the process of enabling individuals and communities to increase control over the determinants of health and thereby improve their health' (WHO 1986). Health promotion as a defined practice is relatively new in comparison to public health, only establishing itself towards the end of the twentieth century. A series of health promotion charters have been created, stating the guiding principles of health promotion, perhaps the most significant being the Ottawa Charter of 1986. Key points in this charter were:

- Creating healthy public policy, so that laws passed, taxation levied and guidelines and standards set by national and local government should take account of and strive to improve health.
- Creating supportive environments to improve health so people live in safe and satisfying environments which protect natural resources.
- Strengthening community action by encouraging people to engage in health both for their community and themselves.
- Developing the personal skills of individuals so that they will have the information and skills to make informed decisions about their health and cope with health issues they face.
- Reorienting health services from illness services to services which focus more on the prevention of disease and the promotion of well-being.

(WHO 1986)

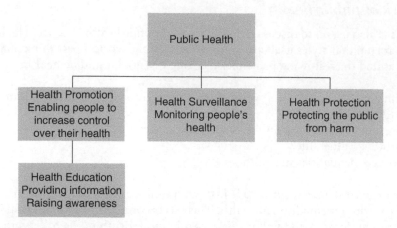

**Figure 1.1** The work of public health

Health education, informing and raising awareness of health issues is a vital first step in promoting health. It is essential for people to know the risks of certain behaviours, for example, before they can be expected to change this behaviour. At first sight the principles of health promotion don't seem too different from those of public health and there is certainly overlap, if not a little rivalry. The important thing is not to get carried away by semantics.

Figure 1.1 probably best explains how the different strands of public health work together.

## The growth and changing nature of public health

Throughout history people have sought ways to limit ill health and the spread of disease. During the plague people carried around oranges studded with pungent spices such as cloves thinking that in warding away the smell of disease the disease itself would be kept at bay. This is because until the nineteenth century causes of disease and methods of transmission were largely unknown. A common belief was the miasma theory, which had dominated for centuries and was based on the notion that contaminated air was responsible for spreading disease. This theory was superseded by germ theory once microorganisms were proved to be responsible for infectious disease. The birth of the modern public health movement arose out of this discovery and the need to combat the appalling number of deaths caused by infection. Before the days of antibiotics, which were not in common usage until after the Second World War, public health measures focused on cleanliness, better housing with less overcrowding, clean water supply and sewage and better nutrition, all of which combined contributed to the dramatic drop in deaths caused by infectious disease. In England and Wales in 1840 there were 70 deaths from measles in every 100,000 of the population (ONS 1997), whereas in 2007 only one child died from measles in the whole of the UK (Health Protection Agency 2012). The trend is the same for all of the common childhood diseases. Medical advances had played their part, widespread vaccination for smallpox was established in the Victorian period and antiseptics were created and used widely. However, as vaccination for most childhood illnesses and other diseases such as tuberculosis were not available until the later part of the twentieth century, it is the improved living conditions aided by widespread improvement in standard of living over this period that should take the credit for this change (Baggott 2000). Unfortunately, however, the developed world is not wholly free of infectious disease. Overuse of antibiotics has caused microbial resistance and new strains of viruses and bacteria can still cause panic, as seen in the case of the mercifully mild swine flu epidemic of 2009. It is important to stress that improvement in living conditions is an essential first step towards combating infectious disease. In developed nations we have numerous regulations to govern the standards of housing, water supply, food safety and sanitation that we take for granted. However, such standards are not universal in the developing world and many preventable deaths still occur. For example, the World Health Organisation states that too many infant deaths still occur from diarrhoea as a result of poor hygiene around bottle feeding and that if infants were exclusively breast fed for their first six months of life 1 million children's lives would be saved (WHO 2011a). In the developing world infectious disease still causes a third of all deaths, with respiratory infections, diarrhoea, malaria, tuberculosis and HIV being the biggest killers (WHO 2011b). Relatively cheap and cost-effective methods of prevention are available to address these specific health issues, such as provision of insecticide-treated mosquito nets to combat malaria, which have been estimated to reduce malaria deaths in the under-5s by 63 per cent (MRC 2012). Distribution of free condoms to prevent the spread of HIV is also an important preventative measure, although agencies working in this field realise that hand in hand with this is the work that goes into facilitating discussions around sexual health and safe sex within communities, which helps challenge current attitudes and behaviour. In addition, as developing countries join the economic revolution and sections of the society become more affluent, individuals adopt the unhealthy habits of Western nations, smoking and obesity levels increase and with them the burden of chronic diseases such as diabetes and cardiovascular disease prevalent in the developed world. The developing world is therefore said to suffer from a dual burden of disease: that of infectious disease because of poverty and that of chronic disease as the result of affluence.

## Modern-day public health roles in the UK

Within developed nations it is the burden of chronic disease that now accounts for much of the focus of the public health movement. The Health Survey for England in 2005 found that 71 per cent of those over 65 had a chronic illness that limited their activities in some way. The commonest of these diseases are musculoskeletal problems, such as chronic back pain, or arthritis and heart and circulatory problems such as previous heart attacks or high blood pressure, but diabetes was also common (HSCIC 2007). Lifestyle factors play a large part in the acquisition of such diseases; for instance, an unhealthy diet and obesity leads to coronary heart disease and diabetes and also puts excess weight and therefore stress on joints, leading to osteoarthritis. Risk factors will be discussed in more depth in the following chapter, but it is the limiting of these risk factors by providing information and supporting people through lifestyle change that forms much of the work of health promoters working in public health. In addition to combating the growth of chronic disease and reducing health inequalities, the public health workforce has a responsibility to tackle acute problems such as an outbreak of salmonella or meningitis, for example, or on a more global level to work with other nations to prevent pandemics such as influenza and to instigate measures to prevent spread. The public health workforce also responds to emergencies. An all too common problem in recent years in the UK has been flooding. Emergency plans ensure that all services work together and in this instance would provide clean drinking water when supplies have been disrupted and arrange emergency shelters for those affected. Perhaps this public health work is more visible when responding to natural disasters in the third world like drought, tsunamis and earthquakes.

## Who works within public health?

We have already discussed that health is a very diverse topic with many influences which come under the remit of most of society in one way or another. To give a snapshot of those workers who see themselves as directly influencing public health and are probably the readers of this text, see Figure 1.2. The number of workers, both paid and unpaid, who see public health as part of their role is expanding year on year. Public health in

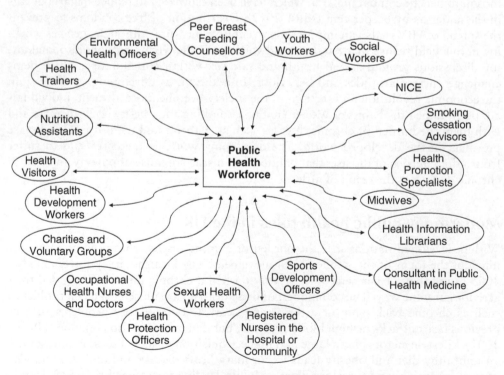

**Figure 1.2** The public health workforce

the UK has now been returned to the place where it began, with the local authorities, who are now charged with commissioning public health services and with leading on local health improvement and prevention. The shift has taken public health commissioning out of the remit of the NHS, which is still focused very much on the diagnosis and treatment of existing disease and is less well placed to address the multiple factors that influence health. Funding is ring-fenced and therefore can only be spent for public health interventions. Decisions regarding priorities and the funding of projects are made at the local authorities' health and well-being boards, comprised of public health services, local councillors, members of the public, GPs and hospital and community health care representatives. In England, Public Health England is an overarching government body that is responsible for national public health priorities such as prevention and screening services, is committed to reducing health inequalities and is also in charge of health protection services. Below this national and local commissioning level are a wide range of grass-roots workers who put into action policies decided at national or local government level. Some workers such as health promotion specialists may work with neighbourhoods to help them set their own priorities and work on specific projects – a toy library or a community garden, for instance. Registered nurses will work more one-to-one with their patients to provide information and support them with self-care and lifestyle change. Youth workers are positive role models who can offer activities and an enjoyable and safe environment for young people, thus enhancing physical and mental health. Community nutrition assistants work in communities and schools to discuss ways of eating healthily and teach cooking skills. Then there is the workforce that is influenced by government priorities but also sets its own agenda – charities such as MIND and Age UK, for instance. Occupational health physicians and nurses are employed by companies and organisations to ensure that the working environment is safe and health promoting. All in all the public health workforce is vast.

## Activity answers

### Unemployment

Limited income gives limited choices in all areas of life and a need to prioritise essentials and cheap alternatives. This affects people's physical health; for example, poor diet and lack of access to structured leisure opportunities and mental health, lack of sense of purpose, decreased self-worth and self-confidence, lack of motivation and depression. These are just a few examples of the ways that unemployment affects health. It has a major detrimental effect on health and causes an increase in ill health and premature death (Wilkinson and Marmot 2003).

### Family

Family attitudes and behaviour influence family members' own attitudes and behaviour – parents influence children and partners influence each other. With regards to health this may be a positive or negative influence. A child of a smoker is more likely to smoke themselves, for instance, often obtaining their early cigarettes from their parents. A recent study estimated that 17,000 children start smoking by the age of 15 each year in the UK as a direct consequence of having parents and/or siblings who smoke (Leonardi-Bee *et al.* 2011). In contrast, a household that values educational attainment is likely to pass on that value to their offspring (Davis-Kean 2005). Family responsibilities are also important. By far the greatest degree of caring happens informally within families, often older people caring for partners or middle-aged children caring for parents. This can have a significant effect on the health of the carers themselves. A report by the Princess Royal Trust for Carers (2011) showed that out of the 6 million registered carers in the UK over half were over 50 and 1.5 million were over 60. Of those surveyed almost 70 per cent said that their caring responsibilities had an adverse effect on their mental health and 65 per cent had a long-term physical health problem themselves. Caring for disabled children or those suffering from serious illness also puts a tremendous strain on family members and relationships. Research has shown that parents with disabled children have higher levels of stress and lower levels of well-being than parents with non-disabled children (Brook 2011). Domestic relationships, if strong and supportive, have a significant positive influence on health. Conversely, unhappy relationships or those containing domestic violence have the opposite effect. Research has shown that partners in an unfulfilling, unsatisfactory relationship are at increased risk of cardiovascular disease and chronic pain (McWilliams and Bailey 2010). Whatever the issue, the problems of family members have ramifications for all those in the family.

## The political system of the country

Politics is closely bound to health care and public health policy. In the UK the health service is a nationalised body run by the government. As the NHS is funded by taxation it is important for the government of the day to show the electorate that it provides value for money and effective practice. Health is a very emotive subject and populations have strong views about priorities and what should be available and what should be paid for privately. The problem is there are obviously differences in opinions and the running of health services is often seen as a political football with different political parties using health care to score points against the opposition. The watch word is reform. The term is synonymous with change, but continuous change is unsettling and costs money in itself. Each restructuring is said to cost at least two years of progress in health care provision (Edwards 2011). This drive to change is true around the world, not just in the UK health care system. In stable political systems such as those operating in the developed world, health care systems, despite differences in operation, are largely available to the majority of the population of the country. However, in poorer developing nations provision, especially for the poorest, is by no means certain. Public health or health promotion programmes are often seen as the Cinderella end of provision, with the largest pots of funding going to secondary (hospital) treatment and care rather than preventative services.

## War

War is of course closely linked to the political system of the country. At first sight it may seem obvious how war affects the health of a nation – people will be killed and maimed. There are also many indirect effects of war on an individual's health. Death of loved ones causes severe emotional trauma, it can have significant impact on the income of the family and family members may be required to take on additional responsibilities. Wars shatter communities, houses are destroyed and people are displaced. Also in war the nations' resources are redirected to support the war effort and this may mean lack of funding for other things like developments in health care. Infrastructure including roads and railways may be destroyed, sanitation and water supply disrupted and education suffers, with schools often closing due to the perceived danger. Manufacturing output may boom, which leads to a temporary increase in employment, but generally war is very bad news for health (Sidal and Levy 2008).

## Housing standards

In the developed world the standard of housing is regulated and minimum standards have to be in place. This is not true of much of the developing world where the poorest of the population often live in appalling conditions without adequate water supply, correct sanitation security or space. Poor housing in such regions leads to a prevalence of infectious disease and injury. However, Western nations cannot be complacent as poor housing still affects the health of those in developed countries. Overcrowding aids the spread of disease, poor insulation and inefficient heating contribute to winter deaths, poor layout and inadequate safety equipment lead to accidentally injury and deaths in fires. Lack of personal space affects mental health and also children's educational attainment (Hood 2005). Good planning can address these issues. Good ventilation, hardwood flooring and damp-free homes cut down the incidence and severity of asthma, for example. Planned community building which incorporates open spaces, cycle and walking routes, shops and public facilities such as libraries and leisure centres promotes social cohesion and lessens crime (Jacobs 2004).

## Levels of self-confidence

Our level of self-confidence is bound up strongly with our self-efficacy, the belief that we can achieve something. This is especially relevant when discussing lifestyle change as we need to believe that we can achieve change before we embark on it. This is a key tenet of the health belief model, which will be discussed in more detail later (Rosenstock *et al.* 1988). Self-confidence can also contribute to assertiveness; those with self-confidence are more likely to seek out useful information from others, join support groups, speak their mind and be more proactive. They are more likely to complain to seek redress, be of a stable personality and therefore less defensive or aggressive, all of which leads to engagement in society and good mental health (MacInnes 2006).

## Driving a car

Owning a car and being able to drive certainly gives independence, it saves time in busy modern lives and is convenient. It can be argued, however, that the high level of car ownership is actually driving the pace of life. People no longer need to work near to where they live so that that they can walk or cycle to work and come home at lunchtime. Cars can cause individuals stress, cause pollution, increase death and injury on the roads, limit physical activity and contribute to obesity (IFS 2012). Unfortunately the economic systems of developed countries and increasingly those of developing nations have bought into this way of life with increasing gusto over the last hundred years. A significant shift will need to take place throughout the world for individualised motor transport to give way to shared public transport as people appear to be wedded to their cars. In the UK, for instance, a quarter of all car journeys are for less than two miles, so there should be the possibility that individuals can limit their car use and use alternative forms of transport in some circumstances. Governments around the world are considering ways to limit car use, however the situation is complex. Taxation is a common measure used, but a 10 per cent increase in petrol prices only causes a drop of 1 per cent in vehicle miles in the short term, and as cars become more fuel efficient, taxation revenue from fuel sales is reducing year on year, whereas congestion has been increasing (IFS 2012). Major policy changes such as road pricing may be required to change individual attitudes and behaviour to car use, together with making extensive resources available to make the alternatives attractive enough for people to use regularly.

## Key messages

- Health is socially constructed and people hold differing views on what it is to be healthy.
- Virtually everything in society affects our health to a greater or lesser extent.
- Traditionally, Western societies have failed to acknowledge these wider determinants of health and the medical model has dominated.
- The developed world has largely controlled infectious disease and much of the work of public health now concentrates on limiting chronic diseases such as cardiovascular disease, diabetes and cancer.
- The developing world has both a high incidence of infectious disease and an increasing amount of chronic disease.
- Public health is made up of different aspects: health promotion, health education, health surveillance and health protection.
- Very many people are involved in public health either directly or indirectly, whether they work for local authorities or the NHS, charitable institutions or private organisations.

## References

Arber, S. and Cooper, H. (2000) 'Gender and inequalities in health across the lifecourse', in E. Annandale and K. Hunt (eds) *Gender Inequalities in Health*. Buckingham: Open University Press.

Baggott, R. (2000) *Public Health Policy and Politics*. Basingstoke: Palgrave Macmillan.

Barry, A.-M. and Yull, C. (2012) *Understanding the Sociology of Health* (3rd edn). Peterborough: Sage.

Bircher, J. (2005) 'Towards a dynamic definition of health and disease'. *Medicine, Health Care and Philosophy* 8: 335–41.

Blaxter, M. (2004) *Health*. Cambridge: Polity.

Brook, A. (2011) 'Parenting under pressure and the SEN parent'. *Special Educational Needs Magazine*. Available online: http://www.senmagazine.co.uk/articles/404-parenting-under-pressure-stress-and-the-sen-parent.html.

Cohen, D. (2009) 'Men need primary care at work, debate hears'. *British Medical Journal* 338: b2471.

Davis-Kean, P.E. (2005) 'The influence of parent education and family income on child achievement: The indirect role of parental expectations and the home environment'. *Journal of Family Psychology* 19: 294–304.

Edwards, N. (2011) 'NHS reform is nothing new'. *Health Service Journal*. Available online: http://m.hsj.co.uk/5031606.article.

Health Protection Agency (2012) *Measles Notification*. Available online: http://www.hpa.org.uk/web/HPAweb&HPAwebStandard/HPAweb_C/1195733835814.

Healthworks (2001) Available online: http://healthworkscollective.com/node?ref=navbar.

Hood, E. (2005) 'Dwelling disparities: How poor housing leads to poor health'. *Environmental Health Perspectives* 113(5): A310–A317.

HSCIC (Health and Social Care Information Centre) (2007) *Health Survey for England*. London: Department of Health.

ICR (Institute of Cancer Research) (2009) *Everyman Campaign*. Available online: http://everyman-campaign.org/.

The Independent (2012) 'Politics and the Paralympics: Voters are against cuts to disability benefits'. Sunday 2nd September 2012. Available online: http://www.independent.co.uk/sport/olympics/paralympics/politics-and-the-paralympics-voters-are-against-cuts-to-disability-benefits-8100742.html.

Institute of Fiscal Studies (2012) 'Taxes on motoring' in *Tax by Design, The Mirrless Review: Reforming the tax system for the 21st century*. Oxford: Oxford University Press.

Jacobs, D. (2004) *Housing and Health: Challenges and opportunities*. WHO International Housing and Health Synposium Vilnius. Lithuania: WHO Europe.

Leonardi-Bee, J., Lisa Jere, M. and Britton, J. (2011) 'Exposure to parental and sibling smoking and the risk of smoking uptake in childhood and adolescence: A systematic review and meta-analysis'. *Thorax International Journal of Respiratory Medicine*. Available online: http://thorax.bmj.com/content/early/2011/02/15/thx.2010.153379.full.

MacInnes, D.L. (2006) 'Self-esteem and self-acceptance: An examination into their relationship and their effect on psychological health'. *Journal of Psychiatric Mental Health Nursing* 13(5): 483–9.

McWilliams, L.A. and Bailey, S.J. (2010) 'Associations between adult attachment ratings and health conditions: Evidence from the National Comorbidity Survey Replication'. *Health Psychology* 29(4): 446–53.

MRC (Medical Research Council) (2012) *Malaria Mosquito Nets*. Available online: http://www.mrc.ac.uk/Achievementsimpact/Storiesofimpact/Mosquitonets/index.htm.

Nettleton, S. (1995) *The Sociology of Health and Illness*. Cambridge: Polity.

NHMRC (National Health and Medical Research Council) (1996) *Promoting the Health of Indigenous Australians: A review of infrastructure support for Aboriginal and Torres Strait Islander health advancement*. Final report and recommendations. Canberra: NHMRC: Part 2: 4.

ODI (Office for Disability Issues) (2012) *The Social Model of Disability*. Available online: http://odi.dwp.gov.uk/about-the-odi/the-social-model.php.

ONS (Office for National Statistics) (1997) *Recorded Mortality in England and Wales.* London: ONS.

ONS (Office for National Statistics) (2005) *Men's Usage of the Health Service, Consultations per Year.* London: ONS.

Princess Royal Trust for Carers (2011) *Always On Call, Always Concerned: A survey of the experiences of older carers.* Glasgow: Princess Royal Trust for Carers.

Rosenstock, I.M., Strecher, V.J. and Becker, M.H. (1988) 'Social learning theory and the health belief model'. *Health Education & Behavior* 15(2): 175–83.

Sidal, V.W. and Levy, B.S. (2008) 'The health impact of war'. *International Journal of Injury Control and Safety Promotion* 15(4): 189–95.

Viseltear, A.J. (1982) 'CEA Winslow and the early years of public health at Yale 1915–1925'. *The Yale Journal of Biology and Medicine* 55: 137–51.

White, A. and Cash, K. (2003) 'The state of men's health across Europe'. *Men's Health Journal* 2(2): 63–5.

WHO (World Health Organisation) (1986) *Ottawa Charter for Health Promotion.* Ottawa: WHO.

WHO (World Health Organisation) (2011a) *Ten Facts on Breast Feeding.* Available online: http://www.who.int/features/factfiles/breastfeeding/en/index.html.

WHO (World Health Organisation) (2011b) *Top Ten Causes of Death.* Available online: http://www.who.int/mediacentre/factsheets/fs310/en/index.html.

Wilkinson, R. and Marmot, M. (eds) (2003) *Social Determinants of Health: The solid facts* (2nd edn). Copenhagen: WHO Regional Office for Europe.

Zola, I.K. (1983) *Missing Pieces: A chronicle of living with a disability.* Philadelphia, PA: Temple University Press.

# 2

# The main killers
## *Susan R. Thompson*

## Life expectancy in the UK

A female child born in 2012 in the UK has an average life expectancy of 82.1 years and can expect to be healthy for around 66 years of their life. A male child born in the same year has a life expectancy of 78.1 years, with a healthy life of around 64 years (ONS 2011). Gradually both healthy life expectancy and actual life expectancy is increasing. Generally those living in England have better health than those living in Wales, who in turn have better health than those living in Northern Ireland. Scotland comes last of all, having the highest all causes mortality rate of all UK countries (ONS 2011). Within England itself there is an obvious north–south divide, with the northern areas of the country having significantly worse health than the southern areas (see Table 2.1). Causes of death obviously vary depending on age, but also gender. In the under-fives the leading cause of death is congenital abnormalities, which are life-threatening conditions that babies are born with. From 5 to 34 years it is suicide, especially in young men, who are a staggering three and a half times more likely to kill themselves than young women. In this age group especially, again amongst males, road traffic accidents were also a leading cause of death. From 34 to 65 years the leading causes are coronary heart disease (CHD) in men and breast cancer in women, although lung cancer rates were also high in this group. Lung cancer is also high in the over-65s, along with CHD and stroke. When discussing both of these latter conditions, professionals use the term cardiovascular disease (CVD). This prevalence of CVD amongst the older population groups is the reason why so much public health and health promotion work is focused around individual lifestyle change and also societal measures directed at the prevention of CVD. For those over 80 years of age, dementia joins CVD as a leading cause of death, especially in women (ONS 2011). Cancer remains the second biggest killer in the older population groups, with lung cancer the most prevalent for both genders, followed by prostate and colorectal cancer in men and breast and colorectal cancer in women. The good news is that, while cancers rates are actually increasing in the population, due to improved detection and treatment, death rates from cancer are decreasing (ONS 2011).

Table 2.1 All causes mortality rates for the UK for 2009

| UK region | All causes mortality rate per 10,000 population |
|---|---|
| England | 548 |
| Wales | 589 |
| Scotland | 667 |
| Northern Ireland | 591 |
| England – North-West | 624 |
| England – North-East | 616 |
| England – Yorkshire and Humber | 584 |
| England – East Midlands | 558 |
| England – West Midlands | 566 |
| England – East | 508 |
| England – London | 524 |
| England – South-East | 501 |
| England – South-West | 505 |

*Source*: Office for National Statistics (2012).

## Major risk factors

Cancer, coronary heart disease and strokes are closely linked to individual behaviour. There are nine risk factors proven to affect people's chance of developing CVD, and many of these have in addition been found to increase cancer risk and many other disorders.

### High blood pressure (hypertension)

This is by far the most important risk factor for CVD. High blood pressure can damage artery walls and increase the risk of developing blood clots that cause heart attacks and strokes. As high blood pressure has no symptoms it is important especially for those over 40 to have their blood pressure checked every few years. Adults should have a blood pressure of no more than 140 mm Hg systolic over 85 mm Hg diastolic (British Cardiac Society 2005). The British Heart Foundation estimates that 5 million UK citizens have undiagnosed and therefore untreated hypertension (BHF 2013a). Those already diagnosed with high blood pressure need checks at least yearly to ensure the medication prescribed is working effectively to keep it within normal levels (NICE 2013).

### Smoking

Despite year-on-year reduction in smokers, in the UK 21 per cent of men and 20 per cent of women still smoke regularly, with two-thirds of smokers starting before the age of 18 (ONS 2011). Tobacco use is responsible for 1 in 10 deaths worldwide (WHO 2007). Smoking detrimentally affects every organ of the body and is the leading cause of preventable death and disease in the UK. About half of all life-long smokers will die prematurely, and there is no safe level of tobacco use (Doll *et al.* 2004). Smoking is directly responsible for 25 per cent of all cancer deaths and a major cause of high blood pressure (ASH 2013).

## High blood cholesterol

Having a high level of circulating blood cholesterol causes fatty deposits to form in arteries, narrowing them and therefore making them susceptible to being blocked by blood clots, causing a heart attack or stroke. Levels of blood cholesterol are partly caused by a diet high in saturated fat (for example, from meat and dairy products) and also by levels of cholesterol produced by the body itself in the liver. Some people produce excessive amounts of blood cholesterol regardless of their diet and there is a genetic link to this so it is common in some families (Bhatnagar *et al.* 2008). Having a diet low in saturated fat and increasing exercise have been shown to reduce cholesterol levels. It is also important for adults to have regular cholesterol checks. UK guidelines suggest that adults have a total cholesterol level or 5 mmol/litre or below with a low density lipoprotein (LDL) level of no more than 2 mmol/litre. LDL, sometimes referred to as the 'bad' cholesterol, is the cholesterol which creates fatty plaques in the arteries. Studies show that for every 1 mmol/litre reduction in LDL there is a consequent 21 per cent reduction of the risk of having a heart attack or stroke (NICE 2008). Statin medication, which reduces cholesterol levels, has proved a very well tolerated and effective way of reducing the risk of CVD, as well as reducing the risk of another heart attack in those already affected.

## Diabetes

People who have diabetes are two to four times more likely to develop CVD and also to suffer from these conditions at an earlier age than the rest of the population (NIDDK 2013). People with type 2 diabetes also tend to have other risks factors for developing CVD such as obesity, high cholesterol and lack of regular exercise. Hypertension is more than twice as common in people with diabetes as in people with normal blood glucose levels. Uncontrolled regulation of blood sugar causes damage to blood vessels, making them more prone to damage from atherosclerosis and hypertension (World Heart Federation 2013).

## Poor diet

A diet high in saturated fat leads to high circulating cholesterol levels in the blood and increases the formation of fatty plaques in the arteries. A diet poor in fruit and vegetables leads to increased calorie intake from other sources and therefore the risk of obesity. Fruit and vegetables have also shown to have a protective effect against both CVD and cancer, and people are encouraged to eat at least five portions per day (Reddy and Katan 2004). Diets high in salt (above four grams a day), found in quantities in processed food, increase the risk of developing high blood pressure (Reddy and Katan

2004). Diets high in fibre have been proved to reduce cholesterol levels and eating oily fish twice a week has also been shown to reduce rates of CVD (Ignarro *et al.* 2007). Other possible components of diet such as soya products and nuts have been shown to be beneficial, as inclusion of these in the diet means fewer calories are obtained from saturated fat. It also follows that diets high in sugar due to the high concentration of calories in easily consumed small amounts of food can contribute to an increased risk of obesity, as well as tooth decay.

## Lack of exercise

The World Health Organisation (WHO) states that physical inactivity has now become the fourth leading cause of global mortality. It accounts for approximately 21–25 per cent of the breast and colon cancer burden, 27 per cent of diabetes and approximately 30 per cent of CHD (WHO 2010). The UK guidelines on physical activity are taken from the WHO report and state that adults between 19 and 64 years should do 150 minutes or two and a half hours of moderate-intensity activity throughout the week in bursts of 10 minutes or more. Moderate activity is described as that which makes the individual slightly out of breath – brisk walking, cycling or swimming, for instance. Alternatively, they may chose to do 75 minutes or more of vigorous activity such as jogging or team sports (DH 2011). In addition, adults should undertake muscle-building exercise such as carrying shopping or working with weights at least two days a week and generally reduce sedentary behaviour. Children from 5 to 18 years are recommended to under-take at least an hour of moderate to vigorous activity every day and also to undertake muscle-strengthening exercise or sports (DH 2011). Physical activity is beneficial as it maintains energy balance and helps prevent obesity. It also reduces the risk of coronary heart disease and stroke, diabetes, hypertension, colon cancer, breast cancer and depres-sion. Additionally, it has been shown to have both a preventative and therapeutic effect on musculoskeletal disorders such as osteoarthritis, osteoporosis and lower back pain (WHO 2010). There have also been studies looking at whether physical activity is a pro-tective factor for Alzheimer's disease, although so far these have proved inconclusive.

## Obesity

Being overweight affects the health of individuals in a myriad of ways. First, it puts them at risk of hypertension, diabetes and atherosclerosis, which in turn can lead to CVD. Obese individuals can also suffer from sleep apnoea and musculoskeletal problems due to excess wear and tear on joints. Obesity causes erectile dysfunction in men and stress incontinence in women, and many gastrointestinal problems. There is also the issue of psychological and social difficulties caused by altered body image and stigma (NOO 2013). A simple although not entirely foolproof method of measuring obesity is the calculation of a person's body mass index (BMI), the formula for this being $(kg/m^2)$, that is dividing the person's weight in kilograms by the square of their height in metres. The subsequent score places the person in a weight category: underweight = <18.5, normal weight = 18.5–24.9, overweight = 25–29.9, obese = BMI of 30 or greater. The UK has the second highest obesity rates in the world after the USA. In 2011, 26 per cent of the UK adult population was considered to be obese and the figure is set to increase, with rates predicted to rise to 40 per cent by 2030 (Swinburn *et al.* 2011). There is also a growing trend of people who are morbidly obese with BMIs of over 40. This has been shown to reduce lifespan by 8–10 years (NOO 2013). Childhood obesity is also rising. In 2011, 17 per cent of boys and 16 per cent of girls were classed as obese, and many more were classed as being overweight (ICHSC 2012). There has recently been research into ethnic differences regarding the risk of obesity, and as those within the South Asian population run greater risks of developing CVD and diabetes the BMI parameter of obesity for this population group has been set lower at 25 or above (World Heart Federation 2013). Central obesity (waist size) has been shown to influence the risk of developing CHD. High levels of abdominal fat can increase the production of the dangerous LDL cholesterol. For this reason it is recommended that men do not have a waist size of more than 40 inches (102 cm) and women's waist size should be 35 inches (88 cm) or less. For South Asian men and women again the recommended measurements are reduced to 36 inches (90 cm) and 32 inches (80cm) respectively (BHF 2013b).

## Alcohol consumption

Alcohol-related deaths in England and Wales are rising dramatically. In men, during the last ten years deaths that can be directly attributed to alcohol have more than doubled and are approaching 5,000 per year. In women, deaths from alcohol have risen by a thousand and now stand at 2,500 per year (ONS 2012). It is reported that 70 per cent of British men and 55 per cent of British women regularly drink alcohol at least once a week, with 20 per cent of men and 14 per cent of women binge drinking (ONS 2012). The news relating to alcohol and CVD is not all bad; alcohol has been shown to have a protective effect against CVD, possibly by increasing levels of HDL cholesterol and reducing blood clot formation. However, this protective effect only occurs if alcohol is consumed in moderation, that is 1–2 units per day (Ronksley *et al.* 2011). The recommended maximum daily limits are 3–4 units for men and 2–3 units for women. It is also recommended that people have one or two alcohol-free days each week. Regularly exceeding these levels of consumption puts individuals at increased risk of high blood pressure, leading to heart attacks and strokes; mouth and throat cancer; alcoholic liver disease; and breast cancer in women. In addition, those drinking over the recommended levels are more likely to suffer from depression, weight gain (alcohol being high in calories), poor sleep and sexual problems (NHS Choices 2013).

## Stress

Whether long-term or chronic stress increases risk of CVD is still a contentious issue (McCleod *et al.* 2002). It has been suggested that stress may worsen inflammation in coronary arteries, leading to blood clots, and the release of the hormone cortisol, which occurs in stressful situations, has been linked with increased formation of fat in the body (Sher 2005). Being less able to cope with everyday pressures or distressing life events makes individuals less likely to adopt healthy behaviours and more likely to smoke more, drink more alcohol and eat more food, all of which can lead to increased risk of CVD. Depression and social isolation is seen as an independent risk factor for developing CHD, although the mechanism behind this seems unclear (Bunker *et al.*

2003; Van der Kooy *et al.* 2007). Sudden stressful life events have been associated with coronary events such as angina and heart attacks (McCleod *et al.* 2002; Bunker *et al.* 2003). This is probably due to acute stress triggering the stress response, where adrenaline is produced by the body in order to make it ready for either 'fight' or 'flight'. An excess of adrenaline makes the heart beat faster, increases blood pressure and therefore puts a strain on a susceptible individual, which may lead to an acute coronary event. In addition to its possible links with developing CVD, stress has also been linked to worsening skin conditions, inflammatory bowel disease, asthma, chronic fatigue syndrome and even Alzheimer's; however, more research is needed in order for these associations to be proven and for the actual mechanism to be understood. In order to lessen stress, individuals need to be aware of the factors that cause them stress (known as stressors) and take measures to remove or lessen these if possible. Individuals should examine their workload, whether at work or in their home life, be aware of taking too much on and striving too hard. Fostering mutually supportive relationships, undertaking enjoyable activities and taking time to relax and socialise are essential stress relievers. There are many relaxation techniques individuals may like to try, such as listening to soothing music or meditating, to give themselves a period of relaxation each day (Varvogli and Darvirir 2011). Regular exercise and being outdoors can also help as a stress reliever and can also aid sleep.

## Calculating CVD risk

In addition to the preventable risk factors listed are risk factors individuals can do nothing about. These are age, gender and family history. Individuals are more at risk of CVD as they age, men are more prone than women (although after the menopause women's risk equals that of men), and if a close male family member had a heart attack before the age of 55 or if a close female family member had one before the age of 65, other family members are at increased risk. A close family member is defined as a parent or sibling. Physicians, family doctors and nurses use assessment frameworks such as the Joint British Societies Risk Assessment Tool (British Cardiac Society 2005) to gauge an individual's likelihood of developing CVD based on the risk factors they exhibit. The five key risk factors of age, sex, smoking habit, systolic blood pressure and the ratio of total cholesterol to HDL cholesterol are taken into account and a score for that individual is calculated that equates to a percentage risk of he or she developing CVD within the next ten-year period. When this percentage is 20 per cent or above in individuals yet to show symptoms of CVD, lifestyle advice and clinical treatment such as cholesterol-lowering statins and anti-hypertensive medication are offered to reduce this risk (British Cardiac Society 2005). These interventions are also given to those who have diabetes and those with an existing diagnosis of CVD (those with angina, for instance).

## The developing world

The public health needs of developing nations differ substantially from those of developed nations. In the developing world much of the health challenges are a direct result of poverty and poor living conditions, often married with attempts to sustain life in

| Goal | Current status | Actions |
|---|---|---|
| **6. Combat HIV/AIDS, malaria and other diseases**<br>Halt and begin to reverse the spread of HIV/AIDS, malaria and other diseases<br>Universal treatment for sufferers of HIV/AIDS | HIV is the leading cause of death amongst women of child-bearing age. Access to treatment in poorer countries has increased tenfold in 5 years. One-fifth of childhood deaths in sub-Saharan Africa are caused by malaria. TB still prevalent especially amongst those who are HIV-positive. | Distribution and use of anti-malarial medicated mosquito nets. Free access to antiretroviral medication. Education on sexual transmission and condom use. TB screening and treatment programmes. |
| **7. Ensure environmental sustainability**<br>Reverse loss of environmental resources<br>Reduce loss of biodiversity<br>Halve number without access to stable supplies of sanitation and safe drinking water<br>Improve the lives of slum dwellers | Loss of species continuing. Access to drinking water improving but not universal. 2.6 billion people are without access to toilets. Numbers of slum dwellers increasing. | Building of water towers and piping of water to rural areas. Rainwater harvesting tanks. Investment in solar energy. Monitoring of water supply for contaminants. Hygiene education in schools. Systems to reduce carbon dioxide emissions. |
| **8. Develop a global partnership for development**<br>Develop open, non-discriminatory trading system<br>Deal with debt<br>Provide affordable, essential drugs to developing countries<br>Increase access to IT | Developed countries not adhering to targets for assistance to developing countries. Debt burden is decreasing. Only 1 in 6 people in the developing world has access to the internet. | Developed countries importing more from developing countries. Developing countries attracting more foreign investment. Pharmaceutical companies to donate proprietary vaccines to developing countries. Debts swapped for funds to reduce poverty and aid development. |

*Source:* UN Millennium Development Goals: http://www.un.org/millenniumgoals/

whereby the higher up the social scale people are, the better people's health tends to be. It is not a direct comparison between the rich and the poor, but a gradient; that is, those in the middle of the gradient have better health than those below and those at the top have better health than those in the middle (Marmot 2004).

There is a significant difference in the rates of depression between groups in the highest income bracket and those in the lowest, suggesting a direct link with socio-economic status. Research has shown that increased financial strain, poor living conditions and a lack of resources lead to an increase in depression, especially amongst women, although both genders are affected (Lorant *et al.* 2007). Long-term stress related to having a low income is associated with developing depression (Wang *et al.* 2009). There is also evidence that people in the lower socio-economic groups have a poorer recovery rate from depression and do not respond as well to interventions as those in the higher socio-economic groups (Falconnier 2009). The relationship with socio-economic status is compounded by the fact that often people who suffer from depression experience stigma and prejudice towards themselves, which results in them having problems finding and keeping employment. This, in turn, affects income.

Improvements in the environment, good sanitation and clean water, better nutrition, high levels of immunisation and good housing will lead to an improvement in health. However, populations generally don't benefit in equal measure; when universal interventions are applied it is often the better off who benefit disproportionately (Graham 2009). This phenomenon is termed 'health inequality'. This section will look at the extent of health inequalities, their causes and the ramifications for societies. It will then consider what is being done to address this issue and the barriers encountered.

## Commitment to tackling health inequalities

The extent of the differences in the health of various sections of UK society first came to the public's consciousness with the publication of the Black Report (1980). This used health statistics from 1971 to examine the link between social class and health and asked the question: are people poor because they are ill, or ill because they are poor? It found alarming discrepancies. For example, it found that the death rate for manual workers was twice that of professionals and that male infants born into lower working class families were three times as likely to die as male infants born to professional parents. Health can be seen as a political football and ideologies of political parties strongly affect health policy, hence the Black Report, which advocated structural changes in society, was met with some hostility by the incoming Conservative government of Margaret Thatcher (Asthana and Halliday 2006). Little was done in response to create a more equal society, but primary care services were overhauled and given a more defined role in providing preventative services, a key recommendation of the report. However, it was the individual who was seen as the major change agent; the responsibility, it was stated, laid with them, not society. When the Labour government came to power in 1997 typically the emphasis shifted from the individual to society. The new administration set targets to reduce health inequalities and commissioned an independent inquiry into health inequalities, the Acheson Report (1998), another significant report to provide the prevailing picture. This report cited the need to combat poverty; increase income, educational attainment and employment levels; and improve housing, the environment and transport. Rather than concentrating on health services it acknowledged the part that wider determinants of health play in influencing health status, and recommended improving the standard of living of the poorest in society, which it claimed would significantly reduce health inequalities (Acheson 1998). In total, Acheson gave thirty-nine recommendations and acknowledged the importance of concentrating on the health of children and families in order to reduce child poverty. As a result of the Acheson report the government of the day published a raft of policy documents including the white paper *Saving Lives: Our Healthier Nation* (DH 1999), which advocated partnership working across all agencies to tackle health and health inequalities. Targets were set that by 2010 the differences in both regional life expectancy and infant mortality between manual classes and the rest of the population should be reduced by 10 per cent. The main proposals to bring about changes in life expectancy from birth were to tackle the causes of cancer and coronary heart disease, the biggest killers, which are noticeably higher in areas of deprivation. This led to dedicated clinics to help people quit smoking being set up by all health authorities and doctor's surgeries undertaking screening for lifestyle factors related to coronary heart disease and cancer and ensuring better control of hypertension and diabetes. National Service Frameworks were published that provided commissioners of services and providers with up-to-date research and recommendations of best practice needing to be implemented in specific areas of concern such as diabetes, mental health, obesity and coronary heart disease. The goal of reducing infant mortality saw the setting up of Surestart centres – health and social care centres for families of children aged 0–4 years living in deprived areas. It also saw actions to reduce teenage pregnancy with a wave of sexual health clinics and initiatives aimed at young people.

In 2002 the government published its *Cross Cutting Review* (DH 2002), which examined spending on the whole range of government programmes in education, welfare, criminal justice, environment, transport and local government in order to put actions into place to tackle health inequalities. This led to the setting up of neighbourhood renewal funds to aid regeneration in poorer communities.

However, when an update of health inequalities was published in 2009, although the health of the nation had improved generally with life expectancy having increased and infant mortality having fallen in the intervening years, 'the gap between the worst off and the average has not narrowed' and there were still 'persistent inequalities in income, educational achievement, literacy, unemployment, local areas, anti-social behaviour and crime' (DH 2009, p. 1).

One area of health inequality that did appear to be succeeding was a reduction in child poverty. In 1999, the then Prime Minister Tony Blair pledged to 'eradicate child poverty within a generation'. The introduction of child tax credit in 2003 is cited as a significant contributor to this, with 65 per cent more deprived families benefiting from this support compared with those under previous systems (HM Treasury 2004). It was claimed that 60,000 children were taken out of child poverty between 1998 and 2007 (DH 2009). The work to tackle child poverty continues with the 2010 Child Poverty Act, which seeks to eradicate child poverty by 2020 and was voted for by all three main UK parties and made legally binding. This act calls for the establishment of a Child Poverty Commission to advise future governments and set up a three-year action plan (HM Government 2010).

## Household income and health

There is no doubt about it that reducing health inequalities is a complex area involving many factors and influences on health. Some academics have argued, however, that it is the income gap between the rich and the poor in society that is the most significant factor in causing health inequality. The claim that the differences seen in life expectancy between the rich and the poor is directly related to the way that wealth is distributed in society. Wilkinson and Richard, in their book *The Spirit Level* (2010), present statistics which illustrate that countries that have the widest income gaps, such as the USA, Australia and the UK, have more health inequalities in their society than those countries with less of an income gap, such as the Scandinavian countries and Japan. They argue that life expectancy, infant mortality, teenage pregnancy, mental illness, crime, educational attainment and social mobility are directly correlated with the level of income equality. Unequal countries suffer more from social problems; this is seen as being related to relative poverty, which is how the income of the poorest compares with those on middle incomes and also the wealthy. It is suggested that increased income disparity between people in society leads to a lack of trust and involvement in community by those in the lowest income bracket (Wilkinson and Pickett 2002; Putman 2000). Being at the lower income scale in a society that values success and status, it is claimed, leaves people with low self-esteem and feelings of resentment and inferiority (Wilkinson and Pickett 2006). It is also suggested that being at the bottom of society and made to feel disrespected, put down and humiliated triggers more violence in that section of society compared with more affluent sectors. The results of violence itself have serious consequences for both physical and mental health (Gilligan 1996). The worldwide global recession from 2008 onwards had a significant impact on household income. In 2002 the trend in the UK had been a steady year-on-year growth in average income, although the gap between those at the top of the income scale compared with those at the bottom had also been increasing year on year. In 2012 average income levels were shown to have fallen by near-record amounts, initially back to mid-1990s levels (IFS 2012). Incomes of the poorest families had fallen less than the incomes of middle earners, which in turn fell less than those in the highest income bracket, whose incomes fell by over 5 per cent (IFS 2012). This has resulted in a slight narrowing of the persistent income gap between the rich and the poor, although it is probable that benefit cuts for the poor and tax cuts for those earning over £150,000 per year will see this gap widening again; much depends on the level of economic growth.

## Status and health inequality

Some academics have suggested that the link between poverty and ill health is also to do with the level of control people have over their lives. People who have low status tend to have less control and greater stress. It has been suggested that those who experience or perceive that they are a victim of working hard for little reward tend to have more stress (Marmot 2004). These heightened levels of stress may cause an increase in the levels of the hormone cortisol in the blood stream, which in turn can lead to weight gain and increased susceptibility to illness (Epel *et al.* 2001). In the late 1970s the Whitehall study, a study of over 10,000 UK government workers, showed that it was not executives with higher levels of responsibility and therefore greater perceived stress who were at greater risk of coronary heart disease, as previously thought, but those at the bottom of the organisation. Later the Whitehall II study took things further and sought to examine more closely the links between stress, social position and disease (Cabinet Office 2004). The study found that it was the employees who had unrewarding yet pressurised jobs and who had little control over their workload who had a higher chance of developing coronary heart disease and not those who were allowed more flexibility, held more power and had a higher status in the organisation. This study showed a social gradient of health for a range of different diseases: heart disease, some cancers, chronic lung disease, gastrointestinal disease, depression, suicide, sickness absence, back pain and general feelings of ill health. That is, the lower the job holder's position in the workforce, the more likely they were to suffer from the above morbidities; this despite the fact that Whitehall employees are not counted as amongst the nation's poor. The social gradient of health applies throughout society. The more affluent also become ill, but the poorest have proportionally worse health. These findings have been confirmed by studies in the USA, Europe and Australasia. There is a clear relationship between social position and mortality for the major causes of death. The report states:

> inequalities in health cannot be divorced from inequalities in society [...] to address inequalities in health it is necessary both to understand how social organisation affects health and to find ways to improve the conditions in which people work and live.
>
> (Cabinet Office 2004, p. 4)

In 2010 Michael Marmot published his updated report into health inequalities. Called *Fair Society, Healthy Lives*, it drew up six main policy objectives that were needed to be fulfilled in order to reduce inequalities in health (Marmot 2010). These were:

1. Give every child the best start in life.
2. Enable all children, young people and adults to maximise their capabilities and have control over their lives.
3. Create fair employment and good work for all.
4. Ensure a healthy standard of living for all.
5. Create and develop healthy and sustainable places and communities.
6. Strengthen the role and impact of ill-health prevention.

The report again advocated the need to tackle the social gradient of health and protect the vulnerable: 'Taking action to reduce inequalities in health does not require a separate health agenda, but action across the whole of society' (Marmot 2010, exec summary, p. 10). The chronic long-term sick are generally either unable to work or have erratic work patterns punctuated by bouts of ill health. Marmot stated that the health gap should be narrowed through a mixture of increased taxation and increased welfare benefits or by reducing pay differentials to become more in line with previous levels. A more equal society, he states, will result in a healthier society. Economic benefits for the whole of society that would result if a reduction in health inequalities were accomplished were stated as increased productivity and tax revenue and lesser sickness benefit payments and treatment costs (Marmot 2010). The need for partnership working across local and national government agencies, the NHS and private and voluntary sectors was stressed in order to achieve widespread joined up delivery of projects and initiatives. Essential to this delivery is the involvement of local people and communities, who should be empowered and supported to take lead roles (Marmot 2010).

The Marmot Review was commissioned in 2008 by the outgoing Labour government and before the UK, along with the rest of the world, slid into a long-term economic recession. There has not appeared to be a great push to establish either income or health equality and it remains to be seen whether the Marmot Report will drift into obscurity as did the previous Black Report. The World Health Organisation notes that it is only in times of greater liberality and affluence that there is a commitment to empowerment and equality (WHO 1999).

## Activity

1. Visit the neighbourhood statistics website at www.neighbourhoodstatistics.gov.uk
2. Access the neighbourhood statistics for where you live and compare them with the neighbourhood statistics for Richmond Upon Thames, Local Authority Area.
3. Answer these questions:

   - Under 'Key Figures for Health and Care', find for both areas:

     ○ the life expectancy from birth of males
     ○ the infant mortality rate per 1,000
     ○ the under-18 conceptions rate per 1,000.

   - Under 'Health and Care', find for both areas:

     ○ the standardised mortality ratio
     ○ the percentage of Year 6 children who are obese.

   - Compare both areas' figures with the national average. How do both areas compare?
   - Looking under 'Key Figures for Economic Deprivation', compare the employment rate and the percentage of benefit claimants for both areas.
   - Compare both areas' figures with the national average. How do both areas compare?
   - As a result of your findings can you see a link between deprivation and ill health?

## Key messages

- Worldwide cardiovascular disease and cancer are the two most common causes of death.
- Individual risk of cardiovascular disease and cancer can be lessened by adopting healthy lifestyles.
- Developing nations have a dual burden of disease, suffering from CVD and cancer but also infectious diseases, high maternal and child mortality and poor living conditions that affect health.
- Although generally life expectancy is increasing worldwide, inequalities in health persist.
- In the UK there is both a north–south divide and an income divide, which means those in poorer areas of the country and with lower incomes have worsening health status than those in wealthier areas and on higher incomes.
- There have been many reports and initiatives aiming to reduce health inequalities, although these have had limited success, and health inequalities still persist in both developing and developed nations.

## References

Acheson, D. (Chair) (1998) *Independent Inquiry into Inequalities of Health*. London: The Stationery Office.

ASH (Action on Smoking and Health) (2013) Website: www.ash.org.uk.

Asthana, S. and Halliday, J. (2006) *What Works in Tackling Health Inequalities: Pathways, policies and practice through the lifecourse*. Bristol: The Policy Press.

Bhatnagar, D., Handrean, S. and Durrington, P. (2008) 'Hypercholesterolaemia and its management'. *British Medical Journal* 337: a993.

BHF (British Heart Foundation) (2013a) *High Blood Pressure*. Available online: http://www.bhf.org.uk/heart-health/conditions/high-blood-pressure.aspx.

BHF (British Heart Foundation) (2013b) *Waist Measurement*. Available online: http://www.bhf.org.uk/bmi/bmi_measurewaist.html.

Black Report (1980) *Inequalities in Health: Report of a research working group*. Chair Sir Douglas Black. London: DHSS.

British Cardiac Society (2005) 'JBS 2: Joint British Societies' guidelines on prevention of cardiovascular disease in clinical practice'. *Heart* 91(supplement no. 5).

Bunker, S., Tonkin, A., Colquhoun, D., Esler, M., Hickie, I., Hunt, D., Jelinek, M., Oldenburg, B., Peach, H., Ruth, D. and Tennant, C. (2003) '"Stress" and coronary heart disease: Psychosocial risk factors'. *Medical Journal of Australia* 178(6): 272–6.

Cabinet Office (2004) *Work Stress and Health: The Whitehall II study*. London: The Cabinet Office.

CSDH (Commission on Social Determinants of Health) (2008) *CSDH Final Report: Closing the gap in a generation: Health equity through action on the social determinants of health*. Geneva: World Health Organization, p. 43.

DH (Department of Health) (1999) *Saving Lives: Our Healthier Nation*. London: The Stationary Office.

DH (Department of Health) (2002) *Tackling Health Inequalities: 2002 cross-cutting review*. London: The Stationary Office.

DH (Department of Health) (2009) *Tackling Health Inequalities: 10 years on, a review of developments in tackling health inequalities in England over the last 10 years.* London: The Stationary Office.

DH (Department of Health) (2011) *Physical Activity Guidelines for Adults (19–64 Years).* Available online: http://www.dh.gov.uk/prod_consum_dh/groups/dh_digitalassets/documents/digitalasset/dh_128145.pdf.

Doll, R., Peto, R., Boreham, J. and Sutherland, I. (2004) 'Mortality in relation to smoking: 50 years' observations on male British doctors'. *British Medical Journal* 328: 1519.

Epel, E., Lapidus, R., McEwen, B. and Brownell, K. (2001) 'Stress may add bite to appetite in women, a laboratory study of stress induced cortisol and eating behaviour'. *Psychoneuroendocrinology* 26(1): 37–49.

Falconnier, L. (2009) 'Socioeconomic status in the treatment of depression'. *American Journal of Orthopsychiatry* 79(2): 148–58.

Gilligan, J. (1996) *Violence: Our deadly epidemic and its causes.* New York: Putnam.

Graham, H. (2009) *Understanding Health Inequalities.* Maidenhead: Open University Press.

HM Government (2010) *Child Poverty Act.* London: The Stationary Office.

HM Treasury (2004) *Child Poverty Review.* London: The Stationary Office.

ICHSC (The NHS Information Centre for Health and Social Care) (2012) *Health Survey for England 2011, Children's BMI, Overweight and Obesity.* Available online: http://www.ic.nhs.uk/searchcatalogue?productid=10149&returnid=1685.

Ignarro, L.J., Balestrieri, M.L. and Napoli, C. (2007) 'Nutrition, physical activity, and cardiovascular disease: An update'. *Cardiovascular Research* 73(2): 326–40.

IIFS (Institute of Fiscal Studies) (2012) *Living Standards, Poverty and Inequalities in the UK 2012.* London: Institute of Fiscal Studies.

Lorant, V., Croux, C., Weich, S., Deliège, D., Mackenbach, J. and Ansseau, M. (2007) 'Depression and socio-economic risk factors: 7-year longitudinal population study'. *British Journal of Psychiatry* 190: 293–8.

McCleod, J., Smith, G.D., Heslop, P., Metcalfe, C., Carroll, D. and Hart, C. (2002) 'Psychological stress and cardiovascular disease: Empirical demonstration of bias in a prospective observational study of Scottish men'. *British Medical Journal* 324: 1247.

Marmot, M. (2004) *The Status Syndrome: How social standing affects our health and longevity.* London: Bloomsbury.

Marmot, M. (2010) *Fair Society, Healthy Lives: Strategic review of health inequalities in England post-2010.* London: Institute of Health Equity.

Neighbourhood Statistics Website. www.neighbourhood.statistics.gov.uk.

NHS Choices (2013) *The Risks of Drinking Too Much.* Available online: http://www.nhs.uk/Livewell/alcohol/Pages/Effectsofalcohol.aspx.

NICE (National Institute for Health and Clinical Excellence) (2008) *Lipid Modification: Cardiovascular risk assessment and the modification of blood lipids for the primary and secondary prevention of cardiovascular disease.* Available online: http://www.nice.org.uk/cg67.

NICE (National Institute for Health and Clinical Excellence) (2013) *Guidance on Management of Hypertension.* http://pathways.nice.org.uk/pathways/hypertension.

NIDDK (National Institute of Diabetes and Digestive and Kidney Diseases) (2013) *Diabetes, Heart Disease, and Stroke.* Available online: http://diabetes.niddk.nih.gov/dm/pubs/stroke/#connection.

NOO (National Obesity Observatory) (2013) *Obesity and Health.* Available online: http://www.noo.org.uk/NOO_about_obesity/obesity_and_health.

ONS (Office for National Statistics) (2011) *Life Expectancy at Birth and at Age 65 by Local Areas in the United Kingdom, 2004–06 to 2008–10.* Newport: Office for National Statistics.

ONS (Office for National Statistics) (2012) *Alcohol-Related Deaths in the United Kingdom, 2011*. Available online: http://www.ons.gov.uk/ons/rel/subnational-health4/alcohol-related-deaths-in-the-united-kingdom/2011/alcohol-related-deaths-in-the-uk--2011.html.

Pickett, K. and Wilkinson, R. (2009) *Health Inequality: Major themes in health and social welfare*. London: Routledge.

Putman, R. (2000) *Bowling Alone: The collapse and revival of American community*. New York: Simon & Schuster.

Reddy, K. and Katan, M. (2004) 'Diet, nutrition and the prevention of hypertension and cardiovascular diseases'. *Public Health Nutrition* 7(1A): 167–86.

Ronksley, P., Brien, S., Turner, B., Mukamal, K. and Ghali, W. (2011) 'Association of alcohol consumption with selected cardiovascular disease outcomes: A systematic review and meta-analysis'. *British Medical Journal* 342: d671.

Sher, L. (2005) 'Type D personality: The heart, stress, and cortisol'. *QJM: An International Journal of Medicine* 98(5): 323–9.

Swinburn, B., Sacks, G. and Hall, K. (2011) 'The global obesity pandemic: Shaped by global drivers and local environments'. *The Lancet* (378)9793: 804–14.

United Nations (2010) *The Millennium Development Goals Report 2010*. UN MDG Database (mdgs.un.org). Available online: http://www.un.org/millenniumgoals/.

Van der Kooy, K., Van Hoot, H., Marwijk, H., Stehouwer, C. and Beekman, A. (2007) 'Depression and the risk for cardiovascular diseases: Systematic review and meta-analysis'. *International Journal of Geriatric Psychiatry* 22(7): 613–26.

Varvogli, L. and Darvirir, C. (2011) 'Stress management techniques: Evidence-based procedures that reduce stress and promote health'. *Health Science Journal* 5(2): 74–89.

Wang, J., Schmitz, N. and Dewa, C. (2009) 'Socioeconomic status and the risk of major depression: The Canadian National Population Health Survey'. *Journal of Epidemiological and Community Health*. Available online: http://jech.bmj.com/content/early/2009/08/13/jech.2009.090910.

WHO (World Health Organisation) (1999) *Healthy Public Policy: WHO health 21 targets 1 and 2*. Copenhagen: WHO Regional Office for Europe.

WHO (World Health Organisation) (2007) *The Ten Leading Causes of Death by Broad Income Group*. Geneva: WHO.

WHO (World Health Organisation) (2010) *Global Strategy on Diet, Physical Activity and Health*. Geneva: WHO.

Wilkinson, R.G. and Pickett, K.E. (2006) 'Income inequality and health: A review and explanation of the evidence'. *Social Science & Medicine* 62(7): 1768–84.

Wilkinson, R. and Richard, G. (2010) *The Spirit Level: Why equality is better for everyone*. London: Penguin.

World Heart Federation (2013) *Diabetes*. Available online: http://www.world-heart-federation.org/cardiovascular-health/cardiovascular-disease-risk-factors/diabetes/.

<table>
</table>

# Approaches and models used to promote health

3

### Susan R. Thompson

So far the discussion has centred around the complex nature of what influences health and how these influences combine to produce inequalities in health. Now it is time to move forward to examine what can be done and is being done to reduce these inequalities and improve the health status of individuals and communities. Much of the work comes under the heading of health promotion. This is described as, 'The process of enabling people to increase control over the determinants of health and thereby improve their health' (WHO 1986). This process obviously needs to take many forms in order to address the range of health influences. Researchers and academics who study health promotion have identified common themes and key aspects that make up the work of health promotion and hence seek to clarify the complex interplay of interventions used in practice. This is with a view to providing those tasked with planning health promotion interventions with information and guidance regarding effective practice. This information is characteristically presented as models or frameworks, often illustrated pictorially to aid understanding. Although many models have been devised, there is much overlap between them, so only a few will be presented.

## Five health promotion approaches

Ewles and Simnett (2003) were two of the earliest researchers to study the new discipline of health promotion. They discerned that in essence there are five approaches or types of intervention that, ideally *in combination*, can be used to bring about improvements in health both at an individual and a population level. These are the following.

### The medical approach

This involves the use of medical or clinical techniques to prevent ill health and to reduce morbidity and premature mortality. Such interventions include health screening and monitoring (blood pressure checking or cervical smear tests, for example). This approach also includes the significant vaccination programmes in place aiming to prevent or limit the severity of a wide range of infectious diseases, from whooping cough to hepatitis. Medication is used to prevent and control existing conditions, to keep them from worsening and causing more severe symptoms and more serious health issues. Controlling diabetes by using insulin to maintain a satisfactory blood-sugar level lessens the risk of diabetic complications and heart disease. This approach can also include surgical interventions and procedures such as the controversial but now common gastric band procedure, which reduces the size of the stomach in order to combat obesity, or angioplasty to widen narrowed coronary arteries, preventing a heart attack.

The medical approach has certainly had its successes. Mass worldwide vaccination against smallpox has resulted in the complete eradication of this devastating disease – a major triumph. The approach lends itself to testing via clinical trials more easily than the other approaches, which occur in a less controlled environment, so the effectiveness of medical interventions can be measured more easily. This credibility means the medical approach attracts greater funding than other more low key interventions and is supported by big business such as the pharmaceutical companies and medical supplies manufacturers. It is generally a very expensive approach: new medication, clinical procedures, laboratory tests and the utilisation of highly trained health professionals and the health service infrastructure are all costly. In the UK, the National Institute for Health and Care Excellence (NICE) carefully weigh up each proposed new intervention to decide whether the costs associated with it are worth the life years to be gained. There comes the problem of managing public demand. Health care is an extremely important political responsibility and governments around the world need to be seen to ensure that it is adequately funded. Well-informed sections of the public are alert to new drugs and procedures and could be a vocal force if services are withdrawn, so it is essential that before interventions are introduced they have proven cost-effectiveness, are available to all and can be sustained long-term. The public are generally very supportive of this approach, although it is seen by some as a quick fix. Why eat a healthy diet, for instance, when, if you have raised cholesterol as a result, you can be prescribed statins to reduce it? Irresponsibility can appear to be rewarded at someone else's expense.

## Immunisation and screening

Immunisations are an extremely effective way of combating the spread of infectious disease throughout populations; however, in order to have a significant effect on the incidence of disease at a population level, a significant amount of people need to be immunised. Low take-up of vaccinations prevent this population effect and lead to epidemics. This has been seen in recent years by the outbreaks of measles in the UK, following scares around the measles, mumps and rubella (MMR) vaccination. Screening is an aspect of the medical approach that has expanded in recent years, benefiting from research into the causes and markers of disease. Screening is now possible for a range of conditions throughout the life cycle, from screening of babies for Down's syndrome and cystic fibrosis, through breast and cervical screening, bowel cancer screening and the risk of developing an aortic aneurysm. Screening procedures vary in their level of invasiveness, from a heel prick in babies to a mammogram in older women, but in order to be cost-effective and to encourage uptake, screening needs to be specific, sensitive and safe. Specificity means that it should identify only those with the disease; it should not wrongly identify that someone has the disease when they do not. Sensitivity means that the screening should identify all those with the disease; it shouldn't miss anyone out. Importantly, screening should be safe; that is, it shouldn't cause problems for the individual, either through unnecessary anxiety or physical issues caused by the screening process. The NHS in England has rejected a nationwide screening test for prostate cancer as the test is not specific enough, with two out of three men showing a positive result following the test and then not actually being shown to have cancer after further tests are carried out. The test also proved to lack sensitivity in the fact that it misses men with prostate cancer (London NHS Cancer Screening Programmes 2009). In 2012, research showed that although mammography for breast cancer saved the lives of 1,300 women, an estimated 4,000 women probably underwent unnecessary chemotherapy and radiotherapy treatment for cancers that were too slow growing to ever cause them harm (Independent UK Panel on Breast Cancer Screening 2012). Screening remains an extremely useful public health tool and is improving all the time; however, it is important to provide the public with the facts to make sure that they are aware of the pros and cons of entering into screening.

## Behavioural change

This is the approach that is possibly the most familiar and recognisable when thinking about health promotion. The onus in this approach is on individuals to change their behaviour, the behaviour which is deemed as being 'unhealthy' and results in them being classed as 'at risk' of disease or injury or worsening health. Behaviours such as drinking too much alcohol, having unprotected sex, driving recklessly and being inactive are just a few examples from a myriad of behaviours that have been shown to have a negative effect on health status. The world's health systems invest much time and effort in persuading us all to adopt a healthier lifestyle – after all, individuals lessening their risk by changing their behaviour is extremely cost-effective, costing governments little if anything, but potentially resulting in huge cost savings in health care further down the line. The individual benefits too, of course; for example, after quitting smoking, people find that they feel fitter and are able to do more before becoming short of breath, their cough disappears, they have improvements in taste and smell, their hair is shinier and complexion fresher, and they have more money to spend on other things. This is in addition to the reduction in risk of cancer and heart disease that occurs after quitting (ASH 2009). Supporting individuals through behaviour change forms a core element of the roles of various professional and semi-professional health workers such as practice nurses, health visitors, smoking cessation advisers, community nutrition assistants and sexual health workers, but also those who work outside the health service such as sports development officers, youth workers and cycling officers. All such are tasked with facilitating healthy choices, providing information, equipment, helping set group or individual goals and action plans and maintaining ongoing contact in order to support people through change. The development of these skills will be discussed in more detail in later chapters.

Behaviour change is essential if modern society is to combat the burden of disabling long-term conditions such as diabetes, chronic respiratory problems, coronary heart disease and stroke. However, for this approach to work successfully resources do need to be invested in supporting people through lifestyle change. Money needs to be spent on training and paying for advisers, venues and equipment such as carbon monoxide monitors or free condoms, for example. All too often judgemental statements are made against people which result in victim blaming. As has been discussed, behaviour is influenced by many factors, and there needs to be an understanding by all health promoters that the relationship between the individual and the social environment is complex. Helping people to change involves making a proper assessment of the individual's circumstances and finding a plan of action that meets the goals they have set themselves and is achievable for them. Relapse is common and again the reasons for this need to be understood and worked around. As an approach, evaluation of the effectiveness of specific interventions and services can be hard to prove because of the multiple factors at play in any successful or unsuccessful attempt at change. For example, if someone starts smoking again this may be a reflection on the quit smoking service, or the fact that their partner continues to smoke.

## Educational approach

Health education is the imparting of information regarding the causes of ill health and conversely what can be done in order to benefit health. As such, it is an essential first step for individuals and communities wishing to improve their health; after all, if people aren't aware that using a condom protects against sexually transmitted disease, for example, why would they be expected to use one? Health education takes many forms, from leaflets and posters in doctors' surgeries, to articles in magazines and even storylines in soap operas. Health education has the capacity to reach a large number of people. In this age of mass communication, never before have people been so well informed about health and the causes of disease. However, ignorance and misunderstandings persist. The role of health education will be discussed in more detail in Chapter 5, but the main issue with the educational approach is that, although it is an essential first step, it is not an end in itself. Too often inexperienced health promoters feel that all that is required is the presentation to the public of cause and effect and that this will automatically lead individuals to undertake change. That, for example, if someone is aware of healthy levels of alcohol consumption and made aware of the risks associated with excess consumption, logically they will drink within normal limits. This of course is far too simplistic. Unfortunately, behaviour is influenced by many more things than just knowledge, so it is essential to combine the educational approach with other approaches.

## Client-centred or empowerment approach

The aim of this approach is to provide support to enable people and communities to take control of their health and set their own agenda which relates to their own interests and values regarding health. Individuals and community representatives are seen as partners with health promoters, who act as facilitators and provide information, support and possibly help with funding and resources so health priorities can be identified and action plans created to achieve the goals set. What is important within this approach is that it is the community or individual who decides on what the health need is, not the professional. Health promoters are often at the mercy of departmental or government targets to concentrate on a specific health issue; however, imposing a health priority which does not match the perceived need of the client is self-defeating. Telling people what is

needed rarely works. Conversely, working with a client's high motivation towards tackling a specific health issue will undoubtedly be more successful than imposing on them
a health need that the client does not recognise or prioritise. Empowerment is more of
an ethos or a key principle, perhaps, than an approach, a principle of enabling a power
shift from the professional to the client that should underpin all interactions no matter what the health promotion intervention. Empowering people enables them to gain
the knowledge, skills and assertiveness they require to make positive changes happen.
Empowerment can be a long-term process, so there are few quick wins, and evaluation of effectiveness again can be difficult to prove. Empowerment is very much about
the individual or community choosing their own agenda, which means that a variety
of issues may be identified that are often at odds with the national or local agenda. A
community group may feel, for example, that their priority is rejuvenating a piece of
waste ground, possibly to make into a play area, whereas the local health authority's
public health agenda may be to combat the area's high rate of teenage pregnancy, an
issue which may be of little concern to the residents. Widening the agenda can be seen
as having a diluting effect and is the opposite of a concerted, multifaceted campaign pin-
pointed towards one particular health issue that may result in a population-wide effect.
Ways to promote empowerment will be discussed in more detail in later chapters.

## Societal change

This approach moves away from the individual to concentrate on society as a whole.
The aim of the societal change approach is to bring about changes in the physical, social
and economic environment in order to make healthy choices easier for people to make.
The focus is on changing society, developing policies, guidelines and laws that promote
health at local and national levels. As such, individuals are not singled out and changes
are made that tend to affect everyone. The law banning smoking in public places is
such an example. Other examples include food labelling guidelines, pedestrianisation
of town centres, street lighting and fluoridisation of the water supply. People can rarely
opt out of these initiatives; they catch everyone and can directly or indirectly influence behaviour. It is the societal change approach that perhaps best tackles the wider
determinants of health that were discussed in Chapter 1. Societal change initiatives
consist of laws, manufacturer agreements and guidelines for good practice. The Local
Government Act 2000 for the first time made local governments take into account the
impact that their policies and service provision had on health when they were tasked
with promoting economic, social and environmental well-being (UK Parliament 2000).
This responsibility steadily grew, and in 2012 it was the local authorities in England
that were given the job of commissioning health promotion services. This reflects the
acceptance of the wider determinants of health and the role local authorities can play
in this. As the societal change approach does not pinpoint individuals, it avoids victim
blaming, and as it captures everyone it can result in widespread and effective change.
One year on from the law banning smoking in public places in Ireland, 48 per cent of
Irish smokers said that they were more likely to quit because of the ban, and of those
who had quit, 80 per cent said the law had helped them (Fong and Hyland 2006).
Such national changes obviously reach the whole population, but governments need
to be careful as accusations of the state interfering too much with personal choice are

often made. It is important that the public supports proposed public health measures as, if not, the result could be severely disadvantageous to the political party imposing them. Consultations, adequate warning and information about proposed changes and what they mean and extra support put in place to ease people through change are all essential if the public is to concede and conform. In Ireland, one year on, 83 per cent of Irish smokers reported that the smoke-free law was a 'good' or 'very good' thing (Fong and Hyland 2006). In 2014 the UK Parliament made a commitment to ban smoking in private cars when children are present (UK Parliament 2014). This apparent invasion into the privacy of personal space is much more controversial, even if its goal is to protect children from second-hand smoke. However, other countries such as Australia and parts of the USA and Canada have already imposed this ban, and many other countries are seriously debating the issue.

Although these approaches are explained here as separate entities, in practice the approaches are not mutually exclusive. In fact, each approach overlaps with and complements the others. In order for campaigns and projects to be effective it is necessary to harness all approaches and combine them into an effective whole.

## Activity

Considering the five approaches, can you think of interventions for each approach that are used or possibly could be used to tackle the risk factors of coronary heart disease? Examples of such interventions are given in Table 3.1.

Table 3.1 Five approaches used to tackle coronary heart disease

| Approach | Intervention |
| --- | --- |
| Medical | Use of medication to lower cholesterol and blood pressure. Screening for angina. Coronary artery bypass and angioplasty operations. |
| Behavioural | Weight management and stop smoking clinics. Walking groups. |
| Educational | Posters and websites providing information and tips on adopting a healthy lifestyle and signposting people to services. Television advertisements warning of the dangers of second-hand smoke. Articles in magazines and newspapers. |
| Empowerment | Health promoters working with clients to identify and meet their specific health needs; for example, tackling weight loss before smoking, if that is the client's priority. |
| Societal change | Manufacturer agreements limiting the level of salt, sugar and fat in processed food. Investment in footpaths and cycle-to-work schemes. Policies on school playing fields and school meals. |

## Top-down or bottom-up

Studying the approaches referred to above, it can be seen that some approaches are more top-down, that is, in the control of the health professional or the state – the medical and the societal approaches, for example – whereas other approaches are more bottom-up, within the control of the client – the empowerment and behavioural change approaches being the obvious examples. There has been much debate regarding moving from a paternalistic system, whereby clients largely have decisions about their health imposed on them, to a system where people are encouraged to make their own choices about their health (Whitehead and Irvine 2010). In effect, these two opposites coexist within public health. Laws are passed that require total conformity, and at the same time competent health promoters work to help clients pursue action plans they have identified may work for them. A key driver for governments around the world faced with the burden of increasing demands on health care systems is cost. Limiting the demand on health care systems by bringing about changes in individual behaviour that contribute to ill health is more cost-effective than spending money on health care. Most health care systems are in part, if not totally, funded by taxation, and there is always the political push to limit the tax burden on the population (Baggott 2000). The public are unwilling to pay the price of their neighbour's irresponsible lifestyle. As knowledge has grown about the causes of disease, so has blame. Perhaps when someone died of a heart attack in 1870 the community might have been more sympathetic than today, when voices may be heard condemning the individual's obesity, smoking habit or lack of exercise. What is more, people who die early are taken out of the workforce. Those with a chronic illness may not be working and therefore not contributing to the economy either, rather they may be claiming disability benefits. All the above has resulted in governments taking charge and targeting ill health systematically through legislation, industry-wide agreements, health and safety policies, health screening, road traffic controls and a commitment to providing information to the public through websites and advertisement campaigns. There remains, however, the need for health promoters to adopt a bottom-up approach where the focus of intervention is directed by the client rather than the professional. In this the health promoter is often placed in a dilemma – as they are often a government employee, they are largely directed by priorities set by that government. Services are developed with priorities in mind. In the UK, in the first decade of the twenty-first century a tremendous push was instigated to reduce the number of smokers in the population in order to reduce levels of cancer and coronary heart disease. The Department of Health made £138m available over the three years from 2003 to 2006 to set up smoking cessation services nationwide. Workers were trained, premises found, clinics set up and incentives adopted such as free nicotine replacement therapy (DH 2008). It can be inferred that as funding is directed to key target areas, this leaves less money for the priority of individual clients, should those not conform to the target areas. Despite exhortations to staff to work with the priorities of their clients, health promoters are constrained by funding and the limitation of their role. Smoking cessation advisers will have been employed to run a quit smoking clinic with expectations of a certain throughput of clients and success rate. They will have limited training or time to spend with individuals whose

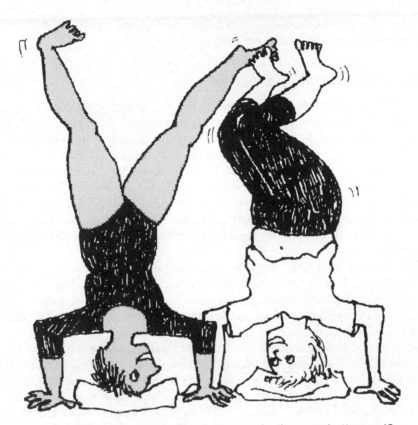

Are you sure that this is what they meant by 'be more bottom up'?

**Figure 3.1** The bottom-up approach

stress level is a fundamental reason why they are unable to quit smoking and no power at all to change the individual circumstances that the client finds themselves in. However, a competent health promoter will realise the limitations of the role and be able to fully assess clients and signpost them on to other specialist services, should they exist. Voluntary and charitable institutions such as Age UK, for example, possibly have more freedom to concentrate on the priorities of their specialist client groups. These organisations often rely partly on government funding but may be able to retain more independence than those working in the public sector.

## Models used in health promotion

As the health promotion movement grew from the 1970s onwards, academics took an interest in studying methods used in health promotion and started to draw conclusions and recommend models of effective practice. These models incorporated the approaches mentioned above and aimed to increase understanding of the complex interplay of methods and ideologies at work via a simplified visual representation.

There are many such models, but there is much overlap and repetition, and only two well-recognised models will be discussed here.

## Beattie's model of health promotion

Beattie's model acknowledged that approaches are either top-down or bottom-up. These he calls authoritative (expert-led) or negotiated (valuing the individual's autonomy). Approaches, he suggests, are also either aimed at individuals or communities. The left-hand side of the model deals with those interventions directed at individuals, whereas the right-hand side looks at more collective interventions. A continuum is used to express these concepts. The continuum is useful as, in practice, approaches blur and overlap, as often does the focus of the intervention. Beattie doesn't use the Ewles and Simnett approaches but identifies four different, yet similar, approaches: health persuasion, legislative action, personal counselling and community development.

Health persuasion is similar, perhaps, to a combination of health education and behavioural change. It is an intervention aimed at individuals and led by professionals. An example is a midwife encouraging a pregnant woman to stop smoking or a poster showing the negative effects of drugs on the body. Health persuasion will be discussed in more detail in later chapters.

Legislative actions are paternalistic or state-directed actions, such as making children travel in the back seat of cars and imposing smoking bans. This equates to Ewles and Simnett's societal change approach, although Beattie, by concentrating on legislative action, ignores the myriad of society-wide agreements and policies, which are in fact much more common than legislative action, which is quite rare. The passing of laws is serious business, hard to reverse and needs a great deal of public support and parliamentary time to enact.

Personal counselling represents client-led interventions and focuses on personal development. In this way it matches the empowerment approach, with the health promoter acting as a facilitator rather than an expert. An example may be an alcohol support worker working with a client to identify his drinking patterns and working together with input from the client to draw up an action plan to limit that drinking to a level that the client feels he can manage to sustain. Personal counselling, if done correctly, is a time-hungry approach. Before clients reach the stage of being able to embark on lifestyle change they may require in-depth and prolonged exploration of past experiences, learned behaviour patterns and efforts to increase self-confidence and self-efficacy. Without these in-depth interventions what can commonly happen is that messages and action plans are just laid over persistent problems and the client is doomed to fail, with the consequent decrease in self-belief that would inevitably accompany this. Personal counselling will be discussed in more detail in later chapters. Community development seeks to empower or enhance the skills of a group or local community. It facilitates community participation and involvement in addressing the needs of communities and can subsequently seek to tackle health inequalities. This may include the formation of neighbour groups to work on specific projects such as a food co-operative, a community garden or a toy library.

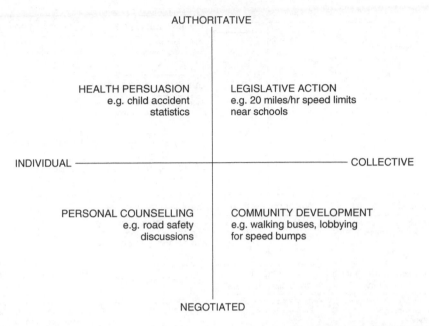

**Figure 3.2** Beattie's (1991) model adapted to show ways of addressing child road safety

Beattie's model uses the four quadrants between the two axes to illustrate how approaches interact with each other and how they are combined. If we take, for example, improving child road safety and preventing accidents as the aim of a series of interventions using different approaches, then Figure 3.2 illustrates the specific interventions that could be used in the relevant quadrant of the model. The quadrant between 'authoritative' and 'individual', which incorporates health persuasion, could encompass local authority child accident statistics collected and given to the parents of children, hence raising awareness of the issue. The quadrant between 'authoritative' and 'collective', incorporating legislation, could consist of an intervention to set 20-miles-per-hour speed limits on roads near schools. The quadrant between 'collective' and 'negotiated', which incorporates community development, could be working with the school community to organise walking buses, where volunteers walk students to school in groups. Setting up a group of interested parents in this way can lead to many interventions; for example, lobbying for speed bumps to slow traffic in the local vicinity. The quadrant between 'negotiated' and 'individual', incorporating personal counselling, could include parents talking with their children about road safety.

## Tones and Tilford's empowerment model of health promotion

The Tones and Tilford (2001) model suggests that health promotion is a combination of health education and healthy public policy. Policies aimed at promoting health will be discussed in more detail later; however, it is important here to define what is meant by healthy public policy. For this it is useful to revisit Winslow's (1923) definition of

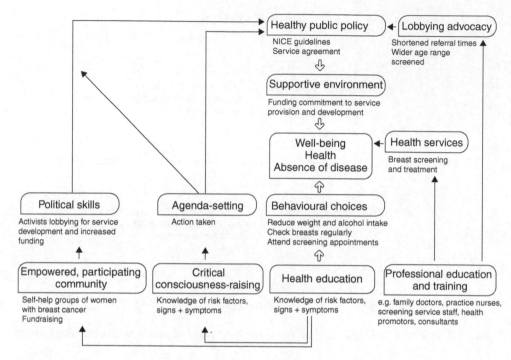

**Figure 3.3** Adaptation of the Tones and Tilford model in regard to breast cancer (2001)

public health, in which he stated that public health interventions were brought about by 'the organised efforts of society'. Healthy public policy is just that – policies, systems, laws, agreements and ways of working put into place that seek to ensure that the health status of individuals and nations is improved, that policies are adopted which enhance health and, very importantly, that policies are not implemented that contribute towards worsening health – in effect, that all policy should be healthy policy. It can be argued, as has been seen in Chapter 1, that due to the wide range of health determinants, all policy has the potential to influence health. However, healthy public policy generally refers to social, environmental, political and economic measures as well as provision of health services and equity of access (Kemm 2001). Tones and Tilford state that health education is the root of all health promotion activity and hence they place health education at the bottom of their model, with all other aspects leading from it. Certainly it is logical that knowledge of the influences on health is essential before changes will be made. Health education, they state, leads to awareness or critical conscious-raising and the setting of agendas to improve health. They also make the leap from health education to the empowerment of individuals and communities. Certainly health education needs to be in place, but there needs to be a lot of work before one naturally leads to the other. Empowerment leads both to the individual adopting a healthier lifestyle and communities lobbying for change. By talking of coalitions they acknowledge the growing movement of partnership working within the field of health promotion, with coalitions of local authorities, health services, community groups, voluntary organisations and business all working together towards similar goals. All the above, they state, forms the bedrock on which healthy public policy is constructed and put into place, which in turn improves health. For local delivery of key policies and guidelines to be effective, it is essential that individuals and local communities are empowered and truly involved in decision-making and implementation (Marmot 2010). Figure 3.3 illustrates how the model may be used with regard to breast cancer prevention and treatment.

By this stage readers may be starting to identify familiar ways of working that they may have become involved in through their work as a health promoter. Nurses may recognise the medical and behavioural approaches and have taken part in these aspects, whereas a health promotion specialist may be more familiar with liaising with local community groups to assess their needs and help them with funding and resources to achieve agreed goals. A health information librarian will recognise their role in providing up-to-date health education material in the form of posters, leaflets, reports, books, and so on, both for professionals and the general public. A youth worker may be involved in working one-to-one with their clients on specific issues, but may also be a part of a wider group lobbying for change or resources for their client group. Whatever the specific role, it is essential to be able to understand the theory and reasons behind adopting certain interventions and also to consider the wider picture of how the public health workforce works together to instigate change.

## Key messages

- There are five main approaches in health promotion.
- Different approaches are used in combination to ensure effectiveness and impact.
- Models of health promotion illustrate how these approaches can work together in practice.
- Health promoters are encouraged to meet the specific agenda of their clients, although this is usually influenced and constrained by policies and funding.
- Health promoters adopt certain approaches and work within parameters according to their specific roles; however, all combine to produce effective health promotion practice.

## References

ASH (Action on Smoking and Health) (2009) *Stopping Smoking: The benefits and aids to quitting.* London: Action on Smoking and Health.

Baggott, R. (2000) *Public Health Policy and Politics.* Basingstoke: Palgrave Macmillan.

Beattie, A. (1991) 'Knowledge and control in health promotion: A test case for social policy and social theory', in J. Gaber, M. Calman and M. Bury (eds) *The Sociology of the Health Service.* London: Routledge.

DH (Department of Health) (2008) *NHS Stop Smoking Services and Nicotine Replacement Therapy.* Available online: http://webarchive.nationalarchives.gov.uk/+/www. dh.gov.uk/en/Publichealth/Healthimprovement/Tobacco/Tobaccogeneralinformation/ DH_4002192.

Ewles, L. and Simnett, I. (2003) *Promoting Health: A practical guide* (5th edn). London: Balliere Tindall.

Fong, G.T. and Hyland, A. (2006) 'Reductions in tobacco smoke pollution and increases in support for smoke-free public places following the implementation of comprehensive smoke-free workplace legislation in the Republic of Ireland: findings from the ITC Ireland/UK Survey'. *Tobacco Control* 15(sup. 3): 51–8.

Independent UK Panel on Breast Cancer Screening (2012) 'The benefits and harms of breast cancer screening: An independent review'. *The Lancet*, 30 October 2012, early online publication: doi: 10.1016/S0140-6736(12)61611-0.

Kemm, J. (2001) 'Health Impact Assessment: A tool for healthy public policy'. *Health Promotion International* 16(1): 79–85.

London NHS Cancer Screening Programmes (2009) *PSA (Prostate Specific Antigen) Testing for Prostate Cancer: An information sheet for men considering a PSA test.* Sheffield: NHS Cancer Screening Programmes.

Marmot (2010) *Fair Society, Healthy Lives: Strategic review of health inequalities in England post-2010.* London: Institute of Health Equity.

Tones, K. and Tilford, S. (2001) Health Promotion: Effectiveness, efficiency and equity (3rd edn). Cheltenham: Nelson Thornes.

UK Parliament (2000) *Local Government Act.* London: UK Parliament.

UK Parliament (2014) Parliamentary Business. Available online: http://www.publications. parliament.uk/pa/ld201314/ldhansrd/text/140129-0002.htm.

Whitehead, D. and Irvine, F. (2010) *Health Promotion and Health Education in Nursing.* Basingstoke: Palgrave Macmillan.

WHO (World Health Organisation) (1986) *Ottawa Charter for Health Promotion: An international conference on health promotion.* Copenhagen: WHO.

Winslow, C.E.A. (1923) *The Evolution and Significance of the Modern Public Health Campaign.* New Haven, CT: Yale University Press.

# 4 Health needs assessment

## Susan R. Thompson

## Definition of health needs assessment

Health needs assessment (HNA) has been described as 'a systematic method of identifying unmet health and health care needs of a population and making changes to meet these unmet needs' (Wright and Kyle 2006, p. 20) or 'a systematic method for reviewing the health needs facing a population leading to agreed health priorities and resource allocation that will improve health and reduce health inequalities' (NICE 2005). Health needs assessment is used to set the policy agenda, plan services and target resources effectively to result in maximum health benefit for both individuals and populations. HNA is conducted at many different levels: internationally, through the work of the World Health Organisation, for instance; nationally, by government health departments; and locally, from hospitals, primary care and local authority organisations right down to neighbourhood groups. Large-scale health needs assessments are carried out by statutory, voluntary, community and private sector organisations such as strategic groups within health and local authority services. Key agencies such as education, transport, local business, leisure, housing, the police and community representatives work together in partnership to agreed goals. Before HNAs are commenced there must be a commitment to addressing a certain issue within a particular target group. These groups may be people with a certain medical condition or commonality, such as asylum seekers or young people or the needs of a certain geographic community or section of the community, for example a workplace or school. It is irresponsible to start an HNA and consult with a client group unless it is expected that something of benefit for that group will come from it. Consultation and involvement raises expectations that should be met, at least in part. This may not be brand new service provision; it may be a service development or alteration to better meet the needs of that group. It is essential, therefore, that key senior managers who can drive through change and direct resources are involved and fully 'on board'. Ideally there should be a project lead who will liaise and coordinate the involvement of key people, consult with the client group, write up the findings and propose an action plan. Consultation may involve meeting with key neighbourhood groups or support groups dealing with a specific issue or meeting with concerned individuals. Other client-based information can be used, such as service evaluations and questionnaires. It is important to make consultation an ongoing process; it should happen at the start of a project to gain an overview, continue at intervals once plans have been formulated and again when plans are in action. Evaluations can then be used to assess whether the initiative or service improvement is actually meeting the clients' needs.

In 2005 NICE advised on a criteria for the selection of issues to form the focus of HNAs. It was advised that the issue ought to be one which, when tackled, would have the most positive impact on health; that is, a determinant of health or medical condition that affects a substantial section of the population. It was also advised that determinants need to be chosen for which effective interventions have been proven in order that a significant difference can be made. The interventions should be acceptable to the client group and would therefore have the potential to achieve maximum impact. Adequate resources should also be made available beforehand to ensure projects may be sustained (NICE 2005). When selecting a priority area to focus on, the effect of the condition on the individuals should also be considered, such as effects on their social role in relationships, as a worker, as a carer, and so on, effects on their level of mobility, whether the condition causes pain or detrimentally affects energy levels or puts the individual at risk of developing mental health problems. These factors may be scored in order to determine the level of negative impact of the condition or determinant under focus (Hooper and Longworth 2002). The selection of priorities for HNAs still remains a very top-down approach, as outlined in Chapter 3, and is heavily influenced by government targets and resources available.

Much of the academic debate around HNA centres on the identification of needs. At a very basic level, the definition of a need is 'the difference between an actual state and a goal' (Liss 1998, p. 9). Whereas clinicians, doctors and nurses, for example, focus on individual patient needs assessment on a one-to-one basis, public health focuses on the health of populations. These populations may be geographically linked – those living in a certain city locality or county, for instance – or, alternatively, sections of a community – young people's health, health of pregnant women or the elderly, for example. Public health also focuses on the needs of groups of people affected by specific health issues, such as diabetes, coronary heart disease or those with mental health problems. These three types of population groupings generally form the focus for health needs assessments of population groups.

## Types of need

A widely recognised description of different types of need was developed by Bradshaw in 1972. He introduced his taxonomy of needs, stating that there were four basic types: normative, felt, expressed and comparative.

### Normative needs

Normative needs are those decided on by professionals. Data is analysed regarding the prevalence of certain conditions and whether or not incidences of those conditions are increasing. Standards are set; for example, the normal blood pressure range. Those people who exceed this range are diagnosed as having high blood pressure and offered medication to lower their blood pressure. They are judged as having a recognisable need in this regard by parameters set by health professionals. Another example is the national UK breast screening programme. The decision to offer three-yearly mammography to women over the age of 50 was arrived at by research weighing up the cost–benefit analysis of offering this nationwide to this age group and not to those under 50. Such large health initiatives are sanctioned by government but others are decided upon and put into place by local health trusts, local authorities and other smaller providers of health and social care. Epidemiology and research provide an essential evidence base for ascertaining normative needs, and these are discussed in more detail below. Normative health needs based on data collection methods are relatively easy to ascertain, although by no means comprehensive, with needs assessment often adopting a narrow disease approach (Kilduff *et al.* 1998).

## Felt needs

Felt needs are discerned by asking clients or patients what their own perceived needs are. These may or may not match what professionals assess people's needs to be. For example, a 55-year-old woman may be unconcerned about her risk of breast cancer, but may state that she needs more respite care for the older relative she is caring for. In her opinion, this is the greater need for her at the present time. It has been said that the most common complaints patients present with to their family doctor are stress, arthritis and chronic indigestion. These have never been identified as priorities formulated in national strategies (Murray and Graham 1995). According to the World Health Organisation, health promotion is carried out 'by' and 'with' people, not 'on' or 'to' people (WHO 1997). In an attempt to discern felt needs, the public is usually consulted before services commence and also when services are in place. Various methods are used to consult with the public – postal questionnaires, small focus groups, community meetings or standing panels – which are representative samples of the population, permanently in place and consulted with on a regular basis. Questions arise regarding consultation: Is it true consultation? Have people been involved from the beginning? Is it a service that they want, or are they being consulted as to the finer points of the service rather than the actual fundamental necessity or structuring of the service? Are people given enough information so that they are able to give informed comments? Who is being consulted with, is it the vocal minority or is it those truly representative of the client group being targeted? Most consultation exercises seem to be one-off events regarding a specific issue, initiated by service providers rather than the public. It is this initiator who generally sets the questions (Jordan *et al.* 1998). There has also been criticism regarding the lack of training in the consultation process, either by those professionals initiating it or for members of the public taking part. Skills in communication, negotiation, compromise, understanding of group dynamics and conflict resolution are all essential skills for people asked to debate emotive issues such as health care, as well as information regarding the specific issue under debate. Felt needs may be better termed as desires, and the public are generally less well informed than professionals regarding the many different pressures on health resources or the level of risk or effectiveness of interventions proposed.

## Expressed needs

Expressed needs are identified by monitoring people's actions using statistics regarding the uptake of services provided. The assumption is that if a service wasn't necessary, it would not be used. For example, if mammography was not popular and women did not attend, there would be poor service uptake and questions would be asked, possibly resulting in closing the service down. However, this is a simplistic reading of the issue. Possibly people turn up at services because they are persuaded that they should do so and are made to feel irresponsible if they do not. Possibly people attend a service because that is the only one on offer, even if they would prefer that the service had a different emphasis. Waiting time for treatment is sometimes cited as an expressed need; however, these needs have usually been judged as being valid by health professionals so could actually be argued to be normative rather than expressed. Use of specific health services also varies between areas, so sometimes reasons why people access a service are hard to quantify. The link between using a particular health service and subsequent improvement in health status is also hard to prove (Wright and Kyle 2006).

## Comparative needs

Comparative needs is the assessment of needs based on what is provided for similar populations elsewhere. This is about addressing inequalities in access to health care and ensuring equal provision for equal needs. For example, one area may have a project providing support to teenage parents, but another area with a similar population of teenage parents does not have a project. This is inequality in health care provision. As we have already seen, much of the work of public health and the health care systems is concentrated on addressing comparative needs.

# Values-driven needs assessment

In an ideal world all needs would be met. However, this is not possible as 'capacity to benefit is always greater than available resources' (Wright and Kyle 2006, p. 21). Health care needs to expand over time. Difficult choices need to be made between fulfilling one need and denying another. Health economists compare costs and benefits, and needs will naturally be prioritised and targeted at those in most need. This involves judgements to be made regarding this prioritisation. Debates focus on who assesses and decides on levels of needs and priorities and what information these are based on and who is involved in decisions that causes the controversy. Within society there is no doubt that judgements are made regarding prioritisation of needs; what might be seen as a need by one person may be seen as an indulgence by another. Needs assessment may be influenced by the organisational agenda, targets and individual professionals' own beliefs and values (Watson 2002). Many factors influence this perception of needs – the quality of the information available regarding a particular issue, the media, the political and economic climate and the cost of interventions, lobbying by pressure groups and the values that exist in society. Health needs assessment is a combination of epidemiological statistical evidence, economics regarding cost versus capacity to benefit and values held by society. The fact that assessment of needs is influenced by the value judgements of the person or organisation making the assessment is an emotive one, but value judgements are made when health care resources are scarce. Rationing of care exists in all health care systems. The National Institute for Health and Care Excellence (NICE) recommends that couples should be entitled to three cycles of in vitro fertilisation treatment, but many primary care trusts do not offer this as other things are prioritised (HFEA 2013). There has been controversy around whether to offer those with alcoholic liver disease liver transplants due to the condition being seen as self-inflicted (Cohen and Benjamin 1991; Lucey 2011).

## Activity

Imagine that you are in the position to decide on health care funding for specific issues or individuals. Below are listed seven separate requests for funding that you have received. Unfortunately you do not possess the resources to fund all of these, so you must choose two.

1. Coronary artery bypass graft for a 72-year-old woman with angina to stop her condition worsening and possibly causing a heart attack.
2. Nicotine replacement therapy – free NRT to those on low incomes to help them quit smoking.
3. Liver transplant for a 57-year-old man with alcoholic liver disease who is now teetotal.
4. Breast feeding peer support programme – continuation of this programme, which has evaluated well and increased the uptake of breast feeding in the local community.
5. Routine inguinal hernia operation for a 36-year-old, otherwise fit man.
6. Chemotherapy for a 9-year-old boy with leukaemia that might possibly cure him.
7. Occupational therapy – funding for an OT to work with adults with learning disability to increase their independence.

In order to decide on which two to fund you may wish to perform quick searches to understand the conditions/interventions in brief. Things you might consider are: the age of the individual(s), the benefit (economic or otherwise) to society, the severity of the issue, the chance of full recovery/success, long-term versus short-term gains and whether the patient is deserving of care.

## Decision-makers

Decisions regarding priorities for funding specific services or interventions, clinical or otherwise, take place on a regular basis within health care bodies. In England, clinical commissioning groups (CCGs) commission most clinical services that take place in hospitals and community settings for all the patients in a particular geographical area. Local authorities have the health improvement/health promotion remit for their locality running; for example, quit smoking services, sexual health services and the myriad of different health promotion initiatives and projects that tackle different health determinants. Public Health England takes the national public health lead, providing resources, directing national campaigns, overseeing public health training and the work of health surveillance and monitoring bodies such as the Public Health Observatories. Health and well-being boards are tasked with performing joint strategic needs assessments (JSNAs) and, as a consequence of these, draw up a joint health and well-being strategy for the locality that sets out goals and action plans for health improvement. The health and well-being board comprises a local councillor, a member of the CCG and representatives from children's services, the local authority public health service and social services, as well as a member of the public health watchdog Healthwatch. However, membership can also include representatives from local charities and voluntary organisations and those who have particular expertise and experience in the public health field. Health and well-being boards have the responsibility of consulting widely both during the JSNA and on proposals contained in the subsequent strategy itself.

The decision to shift responsibility of health promotion services from NHS primary care trusts to local authorities may be a good move as very often health promotion services suffered from being part of the NHS, which is heavily focused on diagnosis and treatment of health conditions and less driven by preventative care. Commonly, health promotion budgets were raided to pay for overspend in other areas such as medication and to reduce waiting times for surgical procedures (Baggott 2000; Entwhistle *et al.* 2007). The health improvement budget for local authorities is ring-fenced (solely to be spent on this) to provide health promotion services, projects and initiatives aimed at improvement in health status and primary prevention, so it should not be sucked away by other demands. Also, as we have seen, a significant number of health determinants are social and environmental and the local authorities, with their remit for providing leisure services, parks and gardens, cycle paths, street lighting, community centres, youth centres, educational provision, housing, play centres and transport, and so on, have the potential to make a significant impact on these determinants. The NHS still has the monopoly on the medical approach to health promotion, outlined in Chapter 3, and CCGs are tasked to work with local authorities in partnership in order to commission joint services. Time will tell if these changes result in the impact required.

## Effective interventions

The HNA should also incorporate an assessment of interventions proposed, their effectiveness and cost-effectiveness. Systematic reviews of interventions used to target specific issues are published by the Cochrane Library and NICE. These reviews take individual pieces of research on specific interventions published in academic journals and analyse them for rigor. A conclusion is then drawn on their effectiveness and recommendations made. Health needs assessment is the first stage in public health or health promotion programme planning, and this and programme evaluation forms the focus of a later chapter.

Health needs assessment should use a combination of information sources in order to obtain a clear picture of the issues for the population concerned. Epidemiological sources of information are available in the form of statistics and research, for example disease rate. This approach is discussed in more detail below. Information then needs to be sought from agencies and organisations regularly in contact with the population group; for example, the range of existing service providers. The felt needs of the population or community under question must be sought to gain information of priorities for that population, what is thought about existing services, what could be improved and what is needed instead (Whitehead and Irvine 2010; Davies and Macdowall 2006). It is important to remember that HNAs can be used to assess a range of services and interventions, not just clinical services, but also community projects and rehabilitation and support services.

## Epidemiology

Epidemiology can be defined as 'the study of the distribution and determinants of disease frequencies in populations' (MacMahon and Trichopoulos 1996, p. 1) or 'the quantitative study of the distribution, determinants and control of disease in populations' (Rose 1992). Epidemiology, therefore, studies the distribution patterns of diseases and their causes and advises on interventions in order to prevent or reduce exposure of the population to these causes, formulating public policy and lobbying for these interventions to be put into place to reduce this exposure. The birth of the modern public health movement probably began with Victorian pioneer John Snow. Snow had been researching outbreaks of cholera in London for some time, trying to establish the cause of these, when in 1854 a serious outbreak occurred in Soho. At that time many physicians and academics thought that smells and foul air transmitted disease. This was termed the miasma theory. However, Snow believed in Pasteur's theory – that microorganisms spread infectious disease. Snow coloured in a map of the houses in the area where people lived who had been affected by cholera and found that all those affected drew their water from one particular street pump. He took the handle off the pump and stopped the epidemic. The experiment then needed repeating in other areas with similar epidemics in order to categorically prove the association. This discovery of the absolute need for a clean, non-contaminated water supply and an efficient sewage system caused the development of London's sewage system and consequently the separation of waste from the water supply, which became a model for other cities worldwide. In the following century public health concentrated mainly on improving environmental conditions; for example, preventing overcrowding, improving sanitation and clearing slum housing to help prevent the spread of infectious disease (Rees 2001). At the time of his experiment, Snow was unsure of the organism causing the cholera outbreak. However, in judging the water to be at fault and then stopping that water from being used he established a fundamental principle of epidemiology. He formulated a hypothesis (contaminated water) and tested it (by removing the pump handle), thus endeavouring to prove causation. In the modern world the gathering of information regarding possible causes of disease, such as examining distribution patterns and determining factors in common and then the experimental testing of interventions, are essential components in both medicine and public health. However, it is still the case that for many conditions the actual mechanism whereby certain factors cause disease is largely unknown. There have been many studies into cot death, for example, and it is now generally accepted that certain factors increase the risk of cot deaths occurring. Cot death is more likely in babies under four months of age, those of low birth weight and those born to mothers under 20 years of age. Cot deaths are associated with babies becoming overheated or when placed on their front or side to sleep, are more common in households that smoke and more deaths occur in winter. Protective factors that have been shown to reduce the risk of cot deaths are breastfeeding and use of dummies (FSID 2013). Nevertheless, although these causal factors have been established, why these factors cause cot deaths is still uncertain. This is not uncommon in the field of public health; evidence is accumulated as to possible causes and effects and further research is undertaken, meanwhile people are advised of these possible links. In the 1950s a revolutionary study proved the link between smoking and lung cancer by studying tobacco use and rates of lung cancer in smokers and non-smokers (Doll and Hill 1950). This, like all good public health research, led to informed public policy, although in the case of smoking the commonality of this behaviour and the political ramifications associated with tobacco control meant that many years went by before effective governmental measures were put in place targeted at reducing smoking levels in the population.

## Epidemiological data

In the modern era epidemiology has access to a range of statistical sources that can contribute to health needs assessment. There is census data, hospital admission rates, cancer registers, index of multiple deprivations scores, employment statistics, surgical operations data, ethnic origin data, emergency department admissions, notifiable diseases registers, to name but a few. Three fundamental measures that are used by public health specialists to chart the course and scope of disease are prevalence and incidence rates and standardised mortality ratios. Prevalence is the proportion of the population that has a disease or condition at a particular point in time (Robinson and Elkan 1996) – for example, the percentage of Sheffield's population who are undergoing renal dialysis for chronic renal failure in Sheffield hospitals at present. Incidence rates deal with new cases (Robinson and Elkan 1996) – for example, the number of UK women who were diagnosed as having breast cancer in 2011. Incidence statistics can be expressed as people at risk of developing a certain condition – for example, if an originally healthy population of 100 is followed for a year, 10 people may be found to have developed arthritis at the end of that year. Therefore, the risk of developing arthritis in a year within the population studied has been found to be 0.1, or 10 per cent. Statistics in epidemiology are of little use unless they are compared with statistics from other areas or population groups – otherwise how would you know that Sheffield has more or less chronic renal failure cases than elsewhere? It also depends on the population studied – arthritis is a disease common in the elderly, therefore a study of 20-year-olds will naturally give different results compared with a study of 60-year-olds. Standardised mortality ratios (SMRs) are used to even up this discrepancy seen in populations so that a true comparison can be made. SMRs compare the actual death rate in a specific population with the expected death rate in that population taking into account the different demographics of that particular population. The standard expected death rate is put at 100, therefore populations that have SMRs over 100 have a higher death rate than expected and those with SMRs below 100 have a lower death rate than expected. This is obviously incremental. For example, a geographical area with a SMR of 50 for breast cancer has half the risk of its women developing breast cancer than the national average. Usually the data is age-adjusted so the differences in the age demographics are taken into account. However, there are many other variables that differ between population groups – gender, ethnic origin and social economic class, for instance – all of which, as we have seen, have an influence on disease. As it is difficult to account for all these variables, a true comparison cannot be made and SMRs remain a blunt instrument, albeit a useful indicator. It is to be stressed that SMRs deal in death only, so incidence and prevalence rates are very important in considering other conditions or issues. Incidence rates are particularly useful for conditions that are short in duration or acute episodes – infectious diseases, for example – whereas prevalence rates are most useful for long-term chronic conditions such as diabetes and asthma. Epidemiological research studies investigate possible factors or determinants that may cause disease. The four common study designs are cross-sectional studies, cohort studies, case control studies and experimental studies.

## Cross-sectional studies

Cross-sectional studies or prevalence studies are one-off, snap shot studies. They divide a population into two and look at a specific factor in relation to the two groups – for example, age of menopause and coronary heart disease in women. One group may be those who reached their menopause before the age of 55, the other group after 55. Rates of CHD for both groups are then accessed and a possible link discovered – for example, women who had an earlier menopause have a greater risk of CHD. Of course, this doesn't necessary prove cause and effect – there may be many other unknown factors which link the women who developed CHD – but it is a starting-point from which to take research further. Cross-sectional studies select study participants, all of whom have a particular disease or condition, and then compare them for certain factors such as level of alcohol intake, smoking status, and so on. These are then compared to a group who do not have that condition and the differences in lifestyle noted. Cross-sectional studies can also be used to assess the success of interventions – for example, what might be the benefit or not for those patients who receive cardiac rehabilitation after a heart attack compared to those who did not. Cross-sectional studies examine factors retrospectively. What was the intervention or factors? What was the result?

## Cohort studies

Cohort or longitudinal studies are prospective. A large group of healthy people are selected, data is taken from them at the start and throughout the study period, they are followed for a number of years and the results in respect to the development of certain conditions are analysed and links made between the development of a certain condition and factors common to those in the cohort who developed this condition. A very famous longitudinal study is the Framington Heart Study in the USA, which made the first links between coronary heart disease and lifestyle by following the population of a Massachusetts town (FHS 2013). There are many modern studies, one of which in the UK, the Breakthrough Generations study, seeks to discover the causes of breast cancer by following 100,000 UK women over a 40-year period (Breakthrough Generations Breast Cancer Study 2013). Both cross-sectional and cohort studies rely on the recruitment of a substantial number of people in order to show up enough results to be statistically significant. They also need to study conditions which are quite common, otherwise the number in the study who develop the condition may be too few to draw any conclusions from.

### Case control studies
Case control studies start with people already diagnosed with the condition under scrutiny and therefore can use fewer numbers and study rarer conditions. This is again a retrospective study and seeks to identify factors common to people with a certain condition and establish possible links.

### Experimental studies
The final category of study is the intervention or experimental study, in which a matched population (one that has as many commonalities as possible, e.g. age group, gender, social class, etc.) is divided into two, with half being given an intervention and half not. This is commonly used in drug treatments, and a randomised controlled trial (RCT) is considered an excellent study design, especially if it is double-blinded. In double-blind trials placebos are used for the group who do not receive an intervention and neither the participant nor the staff administering the intervention are aware of which participant receives what. RCTs are easier for drug treatments. It is more difficult to assess whether physical activity improves mood, for example; after all, people will know whether they are doing physical activity or not, it cannot be hidden from them. However, researchers may be able to divide the group into those doing recommended levels or types of physical activity and those not. There are many issues that can occur with research such as errors in sampling, bias and confounding, which are beyond the remit of this book; however, epidemiological research and statistics and also qualitative research form an important evidence base for health needs assessment if they are analysed properly.

## Risk assessment

The World Health Organisation adheres to epidemiological notions of risk assessment, as well as needs assessment where risk is defined as 'a probability of an adverse health outcome, or a factor that raises this probability' (WHO 2002). Risks can be the probability of contracting a disease, or a factor which raises that risk – for example, unsafe water supply – or a potential that some behaviour has to increase risk – for example, driving too fast puts people more at risk of an accident, and smoking puts them more at risk of lung cancer. More research is still needed into the causes of disease, which is the next step up from making an association. Once an association is made – for example, that sleeping babies on their stomachs increases risk of cot death – research into proving this cause and understanding what is happening in the body to result in cot death is also necessary. Most health resources are directed to treating disease and less is devoted to truly understanding cause. As well as research into risk and the causes of disease it is also important to research protective factors; what can be done to reduce risk. Sometimes these are obvious, for example reducing driving speed, and well known, such as not smoking. However, there are surely many protective factors at the association stage that warrant further investigation to understand the mechanism at work. For example, strong personal relationships have been proved to be a protective factor in reducing morbidity and delayed mortality (WHO 2002), but why this is the case is still largely a matter of conjecture.

## Activity answers

There are no definitive answers to this activity; what is important is the analysis of the decision-making process. What was the thinking behind the choice of your top two most deserving cases? Below is a possible summary of the factors that you took into account when making your decision.

**Inguinal hernia repair** – Usually a straightforward surgical procedure with a high chance of success without complications, relatively cheap, with long-term cure probable. The person is young and therefore has a long, active life ahead of him, during which he will, if fit, be able to contribute positively to society, both economically and socially.

**Liver transplant** – Providing a liver transplant to someone who has damaged their liver through excessive drinking will possibly raise public concerns that the patient is undeserving of resources due to the perceived self-inflicted nature of the problem, although this could be said about many health issues. Does the stigma associated with alcohol addiction generate more public censure than other health complaints? The man has given up drinking and, if he maintains this, the prognosis should be good, but can he 'be trusted' to maintain his abstinence? What support may be available to help him with this?

**Peer support breast feeding** – Breast feeding has been linked to long-term health gains, from an increase in intelligence to reduced infection rates and a decrease in allergies. This intervention has evaluated well so appears to be working. It therefore has a proven track record. Children are the main beneficiaries of this work and many people can be reached by this intervention. However, children do manage perfectly well by being bottle fed, so how necessary is this intervention?

**Coronary artery bypass graft surgery** – This procedure is usually successful in alleviating blockages in the arteries supplying the heart, therefore reducing significantly the risk of the patient having a heart attack and also relieving the patient's angina pain. However, this procedure is fairly expensive and, after all, the patient is already 72 – how much productive life has she got left? Can medication be used instead that will provide quality of life?

**Chemotherapy** – The recipient of care here is a young boy. Society tends to prioritise care for children as they are seen as blameless, having their whole life ahead of them and it being unfair to have it prematurely taken from them. Society emotionally invests in its children to a significant degree. However, chemotherapy can be quite expensive and is it actually going to work? Often chemotherapy only prolongs life for a period of time; will it cure?

**Free nicotine replacement therapy** – Quitting smoking results in significant long-term health benefits to the individual and reduces costs to society in treating diseases linked to smoking. Therefore, isn't funding NRT a good investment? Alternatively, it's the smokers who have decided to smoke, so shouldn't they pay for their own NRT with the money they will save from not smoking? Also, many smokers start smoking again, so isn't free NRT a waste of money?

**Occupational therapy for adults with learning disabilities** – Adults with learning disabilities can gain better quality of life and be less dependent on services, family and carers if they are supported in learning life skills. One OT can work with many people, so isn't this cost-effective? However, how much change can really be made? Will this client group ever be able to get jobs, for instance, and contribute to society?

The discussions above are simplistic and the questions posed play devil's advocate and could possibly be considered as offensive in some cases. The aim is to show a little of the value judgements that are made by society when deciding on who deserves scarce resources. Value judgements are made blatantly in the case of welfare benefit recipients – any vox pop poll by reporters in the street shows this. People may be more reticent in the area of health care, but judgements are still made, even if only privately. There is also evidence of a tug of war between the social model of health, which is often more to do with improving people's lives, and the medical model of health, which often prioritises cure and medical interventions over social interventions.

## Key messages

- Health needs assessment is used to set the policy agenda, plan services and target resources effectively.
- There are different types of need: normative, felt, expressed and comparative. Often normative needs take precedence when undertaking health needs assessment; however, all types of need should be accorded equal weight.
- Epidemiology plays an important part in informing health needs assessment. Disease incidence and prevalence rates can be charted and risk and protective factors associated with certain health issues can be identified.
- Health needs assessments vary in scale and can be conducted by a range of different agencies. Health needs assessments address a particular health issue, or address health issues related to a particular population group.
- Although health needs assessments often originate from departments of health and national priorities, it is important to consult with the target group and people working with that group in order to prioritise goals and gain feedback on ways of working.
- Value judgements are made when deciding on access to health care and public health services. Decision-makers may be influenced by powerful advocates for

particular aspects of care, by public perceptions of priorities in care, by cost-effectiveness of interventions and short- and long-term goals and targets.

# References

Baggott, R. (2000) *Public Health Policy and Politics*. Basingstoke: Palgrave Macmillan.

Bradshaw, J.R. (1972) 'The taxonomy of social need', in G. McLachlan (ed.) *Problems and Progress in Medical Care*. Oxford: Oxford University Press.

Breakthrough Generations Breast Cancer Study (2013) Website: www.breakthrough-generations. org.uk/.

Cohen, C. and Benjamin, M. (1991) 'Alcoholics and liver transplantation: The ethics and social impact committee of the transplant and health policy center'. *Journal of American Medical Association* 265: 1299.

Davies, M. and Macdowall, W. (2006) 'Planning a health promotion intervention', in *Health Promotion Theory*. Maidenhead: Open University Press.

DH (Department of Health) (2011) *The Functions of GP Commissioning Consortia: A working document*. London: Department of Health.

Doll, R. and Hill, A.B. (1950) 'Smoking and carcinoma of the lung'. *British Medical Journal* 221(ii): 739–48.

Entwhistle, T., Darlow, A. and Downe, J. (2007) *Perspectives on Place Shaping and Service Delivery*. Cardiff: Centre for Regional and Local Government and Research, Cardiff University.

FHS (Framingham Heart Study) (2013) Website: http://www.framinghamheartstudy.org/.

FSID (Foundation for the Study of Infant Death) (2013) *Evidence for Reduce the Risk of Cot Death Advice*. Available online: http://fsid.org.uk/page.aspx?pid=682.

HFEA (Human Fertilisation and Embryology Association) (2013) *Fertility Treatment Guidelines*. Available online: http://www.hfea.gov.uk/fertility-treatment-cost-nhs.html.

Hooper, J. and Longworth, P. (2002) *Health Needs Assessment Workbook*. London: Health Development Agency.

Jordan, J., Dowswell, T., Harrison, S., Lilford, R. and Mort, M. (1998) 'Whose priorities? Listening to users and the public'. *British Medical Journal* 316: 1668–70.

Kilduff, A., McKeown, K. and Crowther, A. (1998) 'Health needs assessment in primary care: The evolution of a practical programme approach'. *Public Health* 112: 175–81.

Liss, P.E. (1998) 'Assessing health care need: The conceptual foundation', in S. Baldwin (ed.) *Needs Assessment and Community Care*. Oxford: Butterworth-Heinemann, pp. 9–23.

Lucey, M. (2011) 'Liver transplantation in patients with alcoholic liver disease'. *Liver Transplantation* 17: 751.

MacMahon, B. and Trichopoulos, D. (1996) *Epidemiology: Principles and methods* (2nd edn). Boston, MA: Little, Brown and Company.

Murray, S. and Graham, L. (1995) 'Practice based needs assessment: Use of four methods in a small neighbourhood'. *British Medical Journal* 310: 1443–8.

NICE (National Institute for Clinical Excellence) (2005) *Health Needs Assessment: A practical guide*. London: NICE.

Rees, R. (2001) *Poverty and Public Health*. Oxford: Heinemann.

Robinson, J. and Elkan, R. (1996) *Health Needs Assessment Theory and Practice*. New York: Churchill Livingstone.

Rose, G. (1992) *The Strategy of Preventive Medicine*. Oxford: Oxford University Press.

Watson, M. (2002) 'Normative needs assessment: Is this an appropriate way in which to meet the new public health agenda'. *International Journal of Health Promotion and Education* 40(1): 4–8.

Whitehead, D. and Irvine, F. (2010) *Health Promotion and Health Education in Nursing.* Basingstoke: Palgrave Macmillan.

WHO (World Health Organisation) (1997) 'The Jakarta declaration on leading health promotion into the 21st century'. *Health Promotion International* 12: 261–4.

WHO (World Health Organisation) (2002) 'Defining and assessing risks to health', in *World Health Report 2002: Reducing risks and promoting healthier lives.* Geneva: WHO.

Wright, J. and Kyle, D. (2006) 'Assessing health needs', in D. Pencheon, C. Guest, D. Melzer and J.A. Muir Gray (eds) *Oxford Handbook of Public Health Practice* (2nd edn). Oxford: Oxford University Press.

# 5 Health education and information

## Susan R. Thompson

The World Health Organisation defines health education as 'any combination of learning experiences designed to help individuals and communities improve their health, by increasing their knowledge or influencing their attitudes' (WHO 2013). Health education is an essential first step for health promotion; after all, unless people are aware of cause and effect – that smoking cigarettes, for example, significantly increases the risk of developing lung cancer – why should they think about quitting? During the last century knowledge of the causes of ill health increased dramatically and this led to resources being directed towards the education of the public regarding a multitude of risk factors and the part they play in a range of diseases. The widespread improvement in living conditions and presence of antibiotic therapy has, in the developed world at least, reduced the number, severity and spread of infections. This has caused public health to focus on chronic long-term health conditions that affect longevity and quality of life and are linked to lifestyle factors. Much of the work of health educators is therefore centred around informing people of the nature of these risk factors and helping people with lifestyle change. However, health education is not just focused on helping people avoid the risk factors associated with chronic conditions; health educators also tackle issues such as sexual health, teenage pregnancy, road safety and mental well-being, for instance.

## Health literacy

It is important to note that in order for people to take on board health promotion messages they need to be able to fully understand those messages. In the narrowest sense, being health literate means being able to understand medicine leaflets, follow self-care instructions and appreciate the causes of ill health. There has been much debate around the levels of health literacy in the general population, with studies showing that health information is very often presented in an inaccessible format and presumes an educational level in excess of that of much of the population (Baker *et al.* 1996; Roter *et al.* 1998; Rudd *et al.* 1999). Tables and graphs often present in health information leaflets further compound this inaccessibility. It also follows that information that goes above the heads of the general population will be even more inaccessible for those who do not have the native tongue as their first language or those with a degree of learning disability. Research has shown that the use of symbols and cartoon drawings in health information leaflets significantly increases comprehension (Delp and Jones 1996). Client involvement in the development of materials has also proven to be effective, as has the use of videos, animated cartoons and computer interactive software (Meade *et al.* 1994; Rudd and Comings 1994; Leiner *et al.* 2004). Unfortunately all these are more costly to produce than blank text and require a degree of production expertise, so this may be why many leaflets and other health information resources seem to stubbornly persist in the blank text format. However, if much of the client group these resources are aimed at are unable to access the information, this looks like false economy. This is especially true as inequalities in health mean that the main target group are probably those with low levels of health literacy. Pictorial artwork in the form of symbols and illustrations is a relatively cheap compromise. Pictures should be supported by clear and simple language emphasising key messages and accompanied by links that signpost people on to quality, in-depth information should they wish to pursue this.

Some academics judge health literacy to be wider than a mere understanding of presented information. Nutbeam (2000, p. 262) describes health literacy as 'the personal, cognitive and social skills which determine the ability of individuals to gain access to, understand and use information to promote and maintain good health.' This includes basic knowledge of health services and health determinants, but also the individual's motivation and self-efficacy to pursue healthy behaviours and gain access to services and resources that will aid them in behaviour change. In this way, Nutbeam agrees with the Tones and Tilford model discussed in Chapter 3 that states that health education leads to critical thinking about health and challenging and lobbying for healthy public policy on the part of empowered, health-literate individuals and groups.

## Health education resources

In the early days of health promotion, practitioners were much involved in the distribution of health information to the public. It is still seen as an essential first step in health promotion and individual empowerment. However, it is crucial to remember that providing information is not an end in itself. Health knowledge in developed societies is perhaps greater than ever before, yet, if this is the case, why do these societies have a great burden of preventable disease? Obviously more needs to be done than merely providing people with information, as knowledge of health determinants does not automatically lead to behaviour change, even if that information is accessible to individuals. Health education is just one step in the process towards behaviour change and on its own is relatively ineffective. Individual behaviour is complex and society's influences on this behaviour is very pervasive (Becker 1999). Health promotion campaigns, health fairs, and so on, do have the potential to change attitudes and increase knowledge of certain issues. Posters and leaflets play their part, but they can do little more than raise awareness of an issue and possibly point people in the direction of services regarding that issue. For leaflets and posters to do their limited yet important job they need to be of good quality, widely available and research-based, regarding both content and format, and, crucially, accessible. Optimal formats need to take account of typeface, style, layout, use of white space, positioning of key information, images and language used. Many agencies produce posters and leaflets, and health promotion libraries (see below) are a useful source of these. The very nature of the poster format means that any information conveyed by them must be limited. Posters are found traditionally in doctors' waiting rooms, as such venues, where people are a captive audience with little to do, are considered good places for posters. However, the rise in personal entertainment devices such as iPods and tablets as well as the old fashioned distraction of magazines may cause posters to be ignored. Studies have shown that although posters are read, recall of their content after some time has elapsed is very limited (Ward and Hawthorne 1994; Wicke *et al.* 1994). Nevertheless, there has been some success with using posters as prompts. One project showed that posters positioned in stairwells and lift lobbies were effective at prompting people to use the stairs instead of the lift (Kerr *et al.* 2000). This was possibly because the message conveyed was simple and easy to activate with immediate effect. There are many resources available to health promoters other than leaflets and posters. Visual aids and interactive resources are especially useful for children, the learning disabled and those who struggle with literacy, but they are also more fun and appealing to the public as a whole. It has been well recognised for some time that interactive teaching techniques are much more effective than passive ones such as listening to others or reading (Kolb 1984; Benware 1984). To this end a gambit of 3-D models, board games, computer software and other formats have been produced. These range from visual representations of levels of fat and sugar in certain foodstuffs, to talking mats with interactive playing cards, to dummy alcoholic drinks and unit calculators, and many other resources, which can be purchased or loaned through health information resource libraries.

## Health information resource libraries

Health information resource libraries usually sit within local public health departments and act as an essential one-stop shop for the wider public health workforce. Scattered throughout the UK, not all libraries work to the same model, therefore services provided vary; however, most act as a repository for health promotion text books, government policy documents, leaflets, posters, DVDs, teaching packs, visual aids and models on a wide variety of health issues, some of which can be loaned, some of which are free to take away. Health promoters may be able to access and request resources online via the library's website. Health promotion libraries staffed by qualified librarians can also provide a service more tailored to the needs of the health promoter, performing literature searches and collating up-to-date evidence on and services related to specific health issues. Good libraries have a dedicated budget to purchase new resources and up-to-date textbooks, and routinely review their stock for out-of-date materials. Some provide email bulletins to inform their users of the latest research and service information with regard to public health, ensuring that new developments and research are fed through to the health promotion workforce. As librarians often work alongside health promotion specialists within the public health departments, they are able to liaise with these professionals regarding the best resources to purchase. Librarians act as a quality controller of information, ensuring leaflets are from reputable sources and free from bias. Health promotion libraries tend not to stock leaflets that endorse or advertise particular products. Leaflet topics range from general lifestyle to those related to specific conditions. Leaflets, posters and other resources are sourced from a range of public bodies and charitable institutions who have expertise in a particular field, so having a central repository for such information relieves the health promoter from the need to source and assess these directly themselves. Many libraries act as a repository for campaign materials for nationwide campaigns such as World AIDS Day or National Stop Smoking Day, and are able to issue packs of these materials to health promoters for use at health fairs or events.

## The art of persuasion

In the modern world the public is bombarded with health messages from a range of sources. These messages target the individual with the intention that behaviour is changed in some way and that, as a result, the individual is less at risk of the detrimental consequences of their previous behaviour. This involves the art of persuasion, and in recent years health promoters have sought the expertise of the advertising industry to compile media campaigns involving television adverts, posters, leaflets and social media, which will connect with the target group, get the message across and hopefully achieve behaviour change. A successful early, if unsophisticated, campaign was the UK's Tufty Road Safety Club in the 1960s, which aimed to teach children how to cross the road safely. The Tufty road safety campaign allowed children to join a club, therefore providing a sense of belonging, and used merchandising to help reinforce messages, so there were board games and Tufty and friends character models to buy, all very appealing to children of that era. This ability to connect with the audience is still essential. Target audiences need to be able to relate to the central character in a TV advert, for example, and the material needs to be accessible and engaging. With another target group in another age, the approach is very different. Social media is very popular with teenagers; it is seen as being owned by its users and therefore independent of government or corporate control and is an outlet for free expression. All these facets make it attractive to young people seeking to achieve independence, but don't make it immune from being manipulated to promote interest groups, including those connected with health. The internet cannot be trusted as an unbiased source of information. Researchers have shown that customer reviews are routinely manipulated in order to secure higher sales, for instance (Shay and Pinch 2006; Hu *et al.* 2008). Nevertheless, social media and the internet in general are excellent and inexpensive tools for providing health education to a wide audience.

### Health beliefs and attitudes

In his book *Brave New World*, Aldous Huxley (1932) wrote:

> find some common desire, some widespread unconscious fear or anxiety; think of some way to relate this wish or fear to the product you have to sell; then build a bridge from the dream to the illusion that your product, when purchased, will make the dream come true.

This is the way advertisers sell products. For example, a fear of growing and looking old may result in the production of anti-aging creams, so advertisers then persuade older women that their product will make them look younger. A common desire to be free could be exploited by advertisers of new cars with television images of convertibles driving along deserted mountain roads, alongside waterfalls, giving the impression that with this car your dream will be realised. Advertising messages aim to tap into people's value and belief systems. Beliefs are the knowledge that someone holds about something, like an object or an action – for example, you may believe that eating potatoes makes you fat. A value is similar to a standard we set ourselves – for example, what constitutes a good parent. The combination of our beliefs and values forms our attitudes, and our attitudes may make us change our behaviour. Someone may believe that exercise is beneficial and value the feeling of being fit; that person will then develop a positive attitude to physical activity that may cause him or her to undertake regular exercise. So attitudes can change behaviour, but behaviour also has the capacity to change attitudes. Someone may possibly be reluctant to commence counselling, not believing it to be necessary or valuing its effectiveness. However, in time, attending counselling may prove to be beneficial and therefore that person may change their attitude towards it.

## *Social marketing*

One way in which health promoters are now seeking to alter attitudes and behaviour is through the social marketing approach, which treats the public as potential consumers of health information and targets them using the principles and working practices established in the advertising industry. The approach seeks to influence audience behaviour that benefits society as well as the target audience (Kotler and Lee 2008). Basically, social marketers sell behaviours. The aim is for people to make one of four behaviour changes: to *accept* (or adopt) a positive behaviour, for example taking up jogging; to *reject* the adoption of a detrimental behaviour choice, for example deciding that they will not start smoking; to *modify* an existing behaviour, for example cutting down their alcohol intake; or to *abandon* completely a detrimental health behaviour, for example quitting smoking (Cheng *et al.* 2009). Social marketing has brought the advertisers' knowledge of human psyche to the forefront of health promotion and public health and, perhaps for the first time, placed this insight into the public's needs and desires at the centre of health education. Essential to the social marketing campaign model is audience research (Kotler and Lee 2008). Once the target group is identified, an analysis of that audience, their desires, what makes them tick and what will capture their attention and help them to engage with the message, is determined. Focus groups, surveys and psychological profiling, either online or in person, can help with this and draft campaign materials can be created and piloted with the help of volunteers from that audience. As the campaign continues, audience reaction is monitored and changes made that all add to the final evaluation. Research has been conducted into what makes the perfect message, and academics at McMaster University in Canada have developed a twelve-step checklist of criteria that needs to be present for an effective health promotion message. These include presenting credible evidence from a credible source, making the message clear, using incentives, suggesting easy actions and, interestingly, placing the critical or most important aspect of the message at the start of the message (NCCMT 2010).

## The hard sell

The difficulty with having access to the wealth of information we are bombarded with in the modern world is that people can suffer from information overload and just switch off. Advertisers therefore need to try to understand what appeals to specific client groups and engages their attention. There is a need to stand out from the crowd, which has led advertisers into more sensationalist practices so that their message can be noticed above the noise of other outlets. Health promotion campaigns are no different in this respect and in recent years campaigns have become more hard-hitting in an effort to achieve an impact. Generally, health messages tend to be presented negatively; that is, 'if you don't do this (or don't stop doing that) something awful will happen to you'. Rarely are positive messages used that illustrate what can happen if people change their behaviour and adopt healthier practices. Former smokers could be interviewed regarding the benefits they have seen since they quit. Converts can be very passionate and proud about their achievements, which will come through in interviews. A lady may be shown who declares, 'Well, since I've stopped smoking I've got more energy, my hair is shinier and I can run for the bus!' However, it is more common to see images of people gasping for breath, restricted to their own homes and on oxygen therapy due to respiratory diseases caused by a life of smoking. Such negative campaigning is termed 'fear appeal', and suggests that failure to act on a health message will result in dire consequences for the individual. Fear appeal advertisements aim to connect with their target group so that these individuals are able to relate to the message, see it as relevant to them and also serious enough in its implications to be taken on board. There also needs to be information contained in the ad that individuals can act on in order to negate or reduce their risk (Lennon and Rentfro 2010). These three components of relevance, seriousness and self-efficacy correspond with the health belief model (Rosenstock *et al.* 1988), which will be discussed further in the following chapter. Research shows that presentation of negative consequences of actions tends to grab people's attention, possibly because people are more sensitive to losses than gains (Tversky and Kahneman 1981). However, O'Keefe and Jensen (2008) performed a systematic review looking at gain-framed (positive benefits gained from) versus loss-framed (negative consequences resulting from) message presentation. They failed to prove that loss-framed messages were any more engaging than gain-framed messages. People appeared to be more engaged when the benefits of positive actions for health were presented to them rather than when the key aspect of the message focused on negative consequences of certain actions or inactions. This was especially noticeable when the message focused on the prevention of disease. It was less evident when the message was concerned with screening, possibly because screening has the potential to uncover existing disease, which is an uncomfortable subject for individuals to deal with. The question is why governments, health departments and organisations persist in presenting fear appeal messages when there is little evidence that these result in significant behaviour change. Is it because society seems to have more of a natural predilection for punishment than reward? If so, it is a sad indictment, but one look at health policy leaves the reader in no doubt that this is the case. There are many examples of health legislation to force compliance with healthy behaviours; for example, speed limits, seat belt laws, not smoking in public places and taxation to punish the unhealthy behaviours of drinking and smoking. Less in evidence are incentives to reward people for indulging in healthy behaviours such as eating a healthy diet and undertaking regular physical activity; in fact, these have costs associated with them.

The debate regarding persuasive messages is not a new one. In 1908 two psychologists, Yerkes and Dodson, studied optimal levels of arousal that were associated with optimal levels of performance or behaviour change. Experiments were conducted that subjected people in a study to various stimuli, some of which were at a low level, others more challenging, thereby resulting in higher levels of arousal in these individuals. They found that people responded best to and were most likely to act on messages that were interesting, but not off-putting. If the way that the message was packaged was boring, people didn't remember it. However, if it was too shocking, people blocked it out. There therefore seems to be an ideal level of arousal somewhere in the middle that grabs people's interest without upsetting them. It was this middle level of stimulation that equated with the most instances of behaviour change. Researchers are still testing out the Yerkes–Dodson law in respect to level of stimulus compared with behaviour change and finding the relationship is still proven (Johnson *et al*. 2012).

## The role of the media in health education

In the modern world there is also the question of desensitisation. We are used to upsetting images in the news and entertainment media, therefore in order to grab people's attention images need to be progressively more and more graphic. Possibly the shock factor, rather than being the model of choice, should be used sparingly. One famous historic example of when this approach was used to good effect was during the AIDS 'Don't Die of Ignorance' campaign in the 1980s. At the time little was known about the condition, but the fact that it disproportionally affected the young was a scary notion for society. It was envisaged that this economically active population group would be decimated by a disease with no cure. Such was the fear of an apocalypse that leaflets explaining the disease and precautions to take were delivered to every household in the UK. The issue is that such outlets for health promotion messages are blunt instruments. Advertising hoardings are seen by all who pass them; television adverts are seen by everyone watching that programme at that particular time. The benefits are that the numbers of people reached can be huge, the downside is that the message reaches many people that the message wasn't intended to reach. Old ladies who don't drive tune in and see distressing pictures of children being injured in road traffic accidents caused by speeding drivers; life-long non-smokers see smokers gasping for breath. Complaints made to the advertising standards authority have resulted in some adverts being withdrawn. In 2007 a UK anti-smoking advert that showed people with fish hooks through their lips attracted the largest number of complaints from the public (774) that year and was consequently withdrawn. The advertisement, which implied that smokers were hooked on cigarettes, was shown to have been offensive, frightening and distressing (*The Guardian* 2007). It is important to consider how people respond to health messages. Research has shown that exposure to negative health messages can cause stress. The ability to cope with this exposure varies from individual to individual, but those from lower socio-economic groups are more likely than those from higher socio-economic groups to respond by blocking out the message, or accepting the message but feeling that they do not have the ability or resources to act on it (Iversen and Kraft 2006). It is also important to be truthful when presenting health messages and avoid both sensationalism and censure. Sweeping statements such as 'smoking cannabis will give you schizophrenia' belies people's experience of taking the drug or the knowledge of others who have taken it safely. This leads to public mistrust of the agencies who are presenting this message, and credibility, once lost, is hard to regain.

## Edutainment

Samuel Goldwyn, a famous Hollywood film producer in the 1930s and 1940s, once declared that 'films are for entertainment, messages should be delivered by Western Union' (BBC 2013). Nevertheless, the media industry has the potential to be an important ally in health promotion. The combination of education and entertainment has given rise to the term 'edutainment' to describe when an entertainment programme also seeks to deliver a message to its audience. Examples of this are storylines in soap operas. In Rwanda, literacy rates are low, televisions uncommon, but radios widespread, so a radio soap opera was chosen by a sexual health project to get messages relating to sexual and reproductive health across to its listeners (CIN 2003). Obviously this has to be subtlety done and the storylines need to be credible and entertaining. It is also important to ensure that professionals knowledgeable about the issues involved are consulted regarding scripts and audience reaction sought. In the UK, in 2012 alone three major television soap operas had storylines dealing with anxiety attacks, binge drinking, early onset dementia and gambling and drug addiction (Priory 2012). Such stories generally aim to raise awareness, increase knowledge and de-stigmatise certain issues, as well as providing a human-interest story for viewers. Awareness-raising by the media or celebrities can also serve as a change agent. When Jade Goody, a UK reality TV personality, died of cervical cancer in 2009, Cancer Research UK issued a statement saying:

> Jade's story has raised awareness of cervical cancer which has led to hundreds of thousands of people contacting Cancer Research UK for information on the disease as the number of hits to our website, CancerHelp.org shows. Her legacy will be to help save lives.
>
> (Cancer Research UK 2009)

Most probably as a result of this high-profile event, by October 2009 the number of women aged between 25 and 64 attending for smear tests in the United Kingdom had grown by 12 per cent on the previous year, which reversed the steadily declining trend of previous years. In 2009, 400 more cases of cervical cancer were identified compared with the previous year, a rise of almost 15 per cent (Cancer Research UK 2012), which undoubtedly saved lives due to this earlier detection. Those who stated that they were especially motivated to attend for screening as a direct result of Jade Goody's experience were younger women and those in lower socio-economic groups, in which screening uptake is traditionally the lowest (Marlow et al. 2012). However, the impetus for this trend was not maintained and subsequently numbers of women attending for cervical screening fell from 3.6 million in 2008/9 to 3.3 million in 2009/10, indicating that one in five women are not attending cervical screening (NHS Information Centre 2010). This is disappointing as cervical cancer is preventable. Cervical screening seeks to detect abnormal cells that in time may turn cancerous, therefore treatment can be given before cancer is even present.

## Social media

Social media such as social networking sites and health forums, blogs and message boards are seen as having an increasing role in the dissemination and discussion of health promotion issues. It is estimated that a third of adults use social media to access health information (Hughes 2010) and as such it is anticipated that use of social media will enable health messages to reach a wider audience. Social media such as Twitter or online health forums can gather data from their communities regarding knowledge and opinions of health concerns and test out thoughts regarding possible interventions. This can serve as a way of getting a campaign or brand across and talked about. An example in the UK is the government's Change for Life website and campaign. Specific Facebook pages for people with a common health issue or interest in common, for example parents of autistic children, can be used to disseminate information, and social media can be used to galvanise support and raise awareness and funding for certain issues – fun runs for breast cancer, for instance. However, this is early days and more research needs to be conducted as to the effectiveness of using social media in health promotion (Neiger *et al.* 2012).

## Magazines

Magazine publishing has been expanding in recent years and women's and men's magazines especially often include health articles, which can raise awareness and provide knowledge of health issues. Such magazines deliver a variety of articles on different subjects, but some of these can be conflicting. It is common, for example, to find features for cake baking a few pages on from weight management advice and information about nutritional guidelines rubbing shoulders with fad diets. This can cause more confusion than clarity and also deliver subtle censure regarding lifestyle and role conflicts (Madden and Chamberlain 2004). Women's magazines especially can be very focused on weight control, but tend to provide simplistic, individual-focused solutions, failing to discuss the broader societal issues and causes of obesity (Campo and Mastin 2007), hence closing down as opposed to expanding the debate. Accuracy is also an issue. One US research study looked at seven women's magazines over an eight-year time period for articles relating to breast cancer. It found inaccuracies, especially with regard to age of onset of the disease, suggesting that younger women were more likely to contract the disease than in fact they are (Merino and Gerlach 1999). So magazines can raise awareness of issues and provide signposting to more detailed information; however, like the rest of the media they are in the entertainment, not health, business, and the need to deliver a good story will generally win over complete factual accuracy.

There have been instances of the media scuppering or distorting health promotion messages. In the case of the MMR vaccine scare, Hargreaves *et al.* (2003) found that the inaccurate public knowledge and understanding of the issue directly corresponded with the media reporting of the issue. The news coverage of certain issues therefore has the potential to create moral panics and distrust of health services.

Watch a health information advert, either on TV or the internet, and answer the following questions.

- Is the message positively or negatively portrayed?
- Who do you think the message is aimed at?
- Would the message be inappropriate or even upsetting if viewed by a vulnerable person, e.g. a child? An adult with learning disabilities? Someone with a mental health diagnosis?
- Does the advert provide information?
- Does the advert point the viewer in the direction of services to help them should they decide to act on the message?
- Do you think it raises awareness of the issue?
- Do you think the message is clear?
- Did the message engage with you, or make you switch off?
- Do you think the advert was ethical?

## Ethics

It may be argued that as we have gained more knowledge of health determinants we are less tolerant of those whose unhealthy lifestyle results in a serious health issue. If a man died suddenly of a heart attack in 1890, responses may have been more sympathetic than might be the reaction today, when comments as to his weight, smoking status and lack of physical activity may result in a 'what do you expect' type of attitude. As we have seen so far, knowledge of health determinants does not automatically lead to changes to a healthier lifestyle, and many people do not possess the ability to change. Is it, therefore, ethical to constantly bombard people with health information when they are not in a position to act? Are health promoters merely adding to social injustice by dumping the problem at individuals' doorsteps, especially when society allows smoking, drinking and overeating, yet censures those who do this? The alternative is to restrict information, thereby denying those motivated and capable of change the help to do so. What is needed from health promoters is an intelligent reading of the whole picture and not a simplistic victim blaming approach. Rather than despairing at people's apparent weakness or lack of self-responsibility, health promoters need to develop the capacity, skills and effective techniques to work with individuals seeking to change.

## Key messages

- A wide variety of mechanisms exist for disseminating health information.
- We are all potential health educators. Virtually everyone can informally impart

health messages, but for the wider health and social care workforce it forms an essential part of their role.

- Newspapers, magazines and broadcast entertainment media can aid the dissemination, understanding and discussion of health issues, but their prime incentive is entertainment.
- The public need up-to-date and accurate information regarding health determinants but it is essential to avoid censuring individuals regarding their behaviour choices.
- Health educators need to possess sound knowledge, update this and be able to signpost people on to appropriate services and sources of information.

# References

Baker, D.W., Parker, R.M., Williams, M.V., Pitkin, K., Parikh, N.S., Coates, W. and Mwalimu, I. (1996) 'The health experience of patients with low literacy'. *Archives of Family Medicine* 5: 329–34.

BBC (2013) *The Film Programme*. BBC Radio 4. 18 April 2013. London: BBC.

Becker, H. (1999) 'Informed decision making: An annotated bibliography and systematic review'. *Health Technology Assessment* (3)1. London: NHS R&D HTA Programme.

Benware, C. (1984) 'Quality of learning with an active versus passive motivational set'. *American Educational Research Journal* 21(4): 755–65.

Campo, S. and Mastin, T. (2007) 'Placing the burden on the individual: Overweight and obesity in African American and mainstream women's magazines'. *Health Communication* 22(3): 229–40.

Cancer Research UK (2009) 'Has Jade Goody's death affected people's attitudes to cancer?' Available online: http://scienceblog.cancerresearchuk.org/2009/05/05/has-jade-goody%e2%80%99s-death-affected-people%e2%80%99s-attitudes-to-cancer/.

Cancer Research UK (2012) '"Jade effect" helps save lives as cervical cancer rates rise'. Available online: http://www.cancerresearchuk.org/cancer-info/news/archive/pressrelease/Jade-effect-saves-lives-as-cervical-cancer-rates-rise-2012-06-01.

Cheng, H., Kotler, P. and Lee, N.R. (2009) *Social Marketing for Health: An introduction.* Burlington, MA: Jones and Bartlett.

CIN (Communication Initiative Network) (2003) 'Radio soap for health education: Lessons learnt by Health Unlimited Rwanda 1997–2003'. Available online: http://www.comminit.com/content/radio-soap-health-education-lessons-learnt-health-unlimited-rwanda-1997-2003.

Delp, C. and Jones, J. (1996) 'Communicating information to patients: The use of cartoon illustrations to improve comprehension of instructions'. *Academy of Emergency Medicine* 3(3): 264–70.

*The Guardian* (2007) 'Anti-smoking TV fish hook ads banned'. 16 May 2007.

Hargreaves, I., Thomas, J. and Speers, T. (2003) *Science and the Media: Towards a better map.* London: The Economic and Social Research Council.

Hu, N., Liu Jr., L., Sambamurthy, V. and Chen, B. (2008) *Are Online Reviews Just Noise? The truth, the whole truth, or only the partial truth?* Rochester, NY: Social Science Research Network.

Hughes, A. (2010) *Using Social Media Platforms to Amplify Public Health Messages: An examination of tenets and best practices for communicating with key audiences.* Washington, DC: Ogilvy Washington and the Center for Social Impact Communication, Georgetown University.

Huxley, A. (1932) *Brave New World*. London: Chatto and Windus.

Iversen, C.A. and Kraft, P. (2006) 'Does socio-economic status and health consciousness influence how women respond to health related messages in media?' *Health Education Research* 21(5): 601–10.

Johnson, C., Moreno, J., Regas, K., Tyler, C. and Foreyt, J. (2012) 'The application of the Yerkes–Dodson Law in a childhood weight management program: Examining weight dissatisfaction'. *Journal of Paediatric Psychology* 37(6): 674–9.

Kerr, J., Eves, F. and Carroll, D. (2000) 'Posters can prompt less active people to use the stairs'. *Journal of Epidemiological and Community Health* 54: 942–3.

Kolb, D.A. (1984) *Experiential Learning: Experience as the source of learning and development*. Englewood Cliffs, NJ: Prentice Hall.

Kotler, P. and Lee, N.R. (2008) *Social Marketing: Influencing behaviours for good* (3rd edn). Thousand Oaks, CA: Sage.

Leiner, M., Handel, G. and Williams, D. (2004) 'Patient communication: A multidisplinary approach using animated cartoons'. *Health Education Research* 19(5): 591–5.

Lennon, R. and Rentfro, R. (2010) 'Are young adults fear appeal effectiveness ratings explained by fear arousal, perceived threat and perceived efficacy?' *Innovative Marketing* 6(1): 58–65.

Madden, H. and Chamberlain, K. (2004) 'Nutritional health messages in women's magazines: A conflicted space for women readers'. *Journal of Health Psychology* 9(4): 583–97.

Marino, C. and Gerlach, K.K. (1999) 'An analysis of breast cancer coverage in selected women's magazines, 1987–1995'. *American Journal of Health Promotion* 13(3): 163–70.

Marlow, L.A., Sangha, A., Patnick, J. and Waller, J. (2012) 'The Jade Goody effect: Whose cervical screening decisions were influenced by her story?' *Journal of Medical Screening* 19(4): 184–8.

Meade, C.D., McKinney, W.P. and Barnas, G.P. (1994) 'Educating patients with limited literacy skills: The effectiveness of printed and videotaped materials about colon cancer'. *American Journal of Public Health* 84(1): 119–21.

National Collaborating Centre for Methods and Tools (2010) *Assessing Health Communication Messages*. Hamilton, ON: McMaster University.

Neiger, B., Thackery, R., Van Wegenen, S.A., Hanson, C.L., West, J.H., Barnes, M.D. and Fagen, M.C. (2012) 'Use of social media in health promotion: Purposes, key performance indicators, and evaluation metrics'. *Health Promotion Practice* 13: 159–64.

NHS Information Centre (2010) 'Number of women tested for cervical cancer falls after 2008–9 peak'. Available online: http://www.hscic.gov.uk/news-and-events/news/number-of-women-tested-for-cervical cancer-in-england-falls-after-2008-09-peak-report-shows.

Nutbeam, D. (2000) 'Health literacy as a public health goal: A challenge for contemporary health education and communication strategies into the 21st century'. *Health Promotion International* 15(3): 259–67.

O'Keefe, D.J. and Jensen, J.D. (2008) 'Do loss-framed persuasive messages engender greater message processing than do gain-framed messages? A meta-analytic review'. *Communication Studies* 59(1): 51–61.

Priory (2012) *Priory Expert Praises Soap Mental Illness Storylines*. Available online: http://www.priorygroup.com/latest-from-the-priory-group/item/news/2012/06/12/priory-expert-praises-soap-mental-illnes-storylines.

Rudd, R.E. and Comings, J.P. (1994) 'Learner developed materials: An empowering approach'. *Health Education Quarterly* 21(3): 313–27.

Rudd, R., Moeykens, B.A. and Colton, T.C. (1999) 'Health and literacy: A review of medical and public health literature' in *Review of Adult Learning and Literacy* (Vol. 1). Boston, MA: National Center for the Study of Adult Learning and Literacy.

Rosenstock, I.M., Stretcher, V.J. and Becker, M.H. (1988) 'Social learning theory and the health belief model'. *Health Education Quarterly* 15(2): 175–83.

Roter, D.L., Rudd, R.E. and Comings, J.P. (1998) 'Patient literacy: A barrier to quality care'. *Journal of General Internal Medicine* 13(12): 850–1.

Shay, D. and Pinch, T. (2006) 'Six degrees of reputation: The use and abuse of online review and recommendation systems'. *First Monday* 11(3). Available online: http://journals.uic.edu/ojs/index.php/fm/article/view/1590/1505.

Tversky, A. and Kahneman, D. (1981) 'The framing of decisions and the psychology of choice'. *Science* 211: 453–8.

Ward, K. and Hawthorne, K. (1994) 'Do patients read health promotion posters in the waiting room? A study in one general practice'. *British Journal of General Practice* 44(389): 583–5.

WHO (World Health Organisation) (2013) *Health Education*. Available online: http://www.who.int/topics/health_education/en/.

Wicke, D.M., Lorge, R.E., Coppin, R.J. and Jones, K.P. (1994) 'The effectiveness of waiting room notice-boards as a vehicle for health education'. *Family Practitioner* 11: 292–5.

# Supporting people with behaviour change

## Susan R. Thompson and Mo Almond

## Working with clients one-to-one

Working directly with clients to help them achieve behaviour change is an important part of health promotion and public health work. Nurses working in the community and also in hospital have a role to play working on lifestyle issues, either one-to-one with their patients or with groups of patients. Health promoters with a specialist remit in smoking cessation or drug and alcohol issues, for example, may run groups or one-to-one clinics. To help workers support their clients and patients successfully, a range of techniques and tools have been developed. The important starting point when commencing work with people on behaviour change is to assess the client's level of knowledge regarding health determinants and also their level of motivation for change. The second essential is to act as a facilitator. The health promoter should support their client to set their own agenda and goals, not dictate to them. Not only is this unethical, it doesn't work, as people cannot be made to change unless they want to.

For people to consider behaviour change they need to connect to a health message and see it as relevant to themselves. Sometimes the message only gets through when life circumstances change and the person concerned is able to connect with it on a personal level. Life events can act as a catalyst for behaviour change. This could be a change in someone's personal health, a health scare that could contradict the 'it couldn't happen to me' mentality that we often subconsciously believe. Possibly a non-cancerous breast lump may cause a women to cut down on her alcohol intake and regularly check her breasts for any changes. Other personal issues may be a realisation of our own deterio-rating health – possibly a long-term smoker now notices that he gets out of breath very quickly and therefore decides to quit. Other situations that may spur people on to con-sider behaviour change may be the change in the health of a friend or family member. The presence of a serious health condition so close to home may serve as a wake-up call, especially if that person is of the same age and gender. Another circumstance that may cause people to consider behaviour change may be assuming responsibility for someone else. Prospective new parents may consider stopping smoking, or a pregnant woman may decide not to drink alcohol and to eat more healthily.

## The health belief model

Research has shown that when people are considering change they weigh up the costs and benefits to themselves of making the change. This is the premise of the health belief model (Nutbeam and Harris 2004). This model suggests that, first, people estimate their susceptibility to a problem; if they are indulging in risk-taking behavior, for example, they consider the likelihood of the problem happening to them. This is heavily influenced by an individual's attitude; for example, they may feel that they can still drive fast and they will not be involved in an accident, so they will continue to drive fast as they don't perceive themselves as susceptible. Young people may smoke because they do not perceive heart disease as a threat, at least for them, and they can always quit later. Next, people consider the seriousness of the possible problem, that is, 'If I get this, how life-limiting will this be?' or 'What would this mean for me?' Again, they may decide that the risk is acceptable and continue. Next, people weigh up what they may gain by changing their behaviour compared with what they may lose. It may seem obvious that people will gain more than they would lose by adopting healthy behaviour, but this may not be the case, especially in the short term. It's all to do with

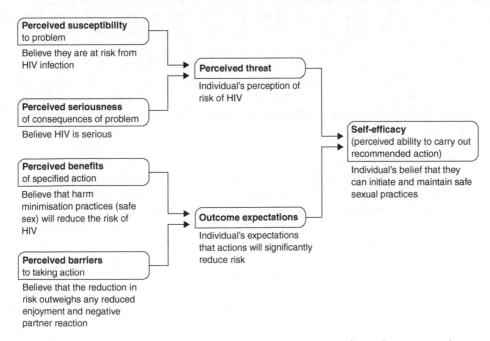

**Figure 6.1** Adaptation of the health belief model (Rosenstock *et al.* 1988) with regard to HIV

the matter of perception. Someone who quits smoking may even in the short term feel fitter, but they will lose their smoking break at work with their mates. It is often this change in social networks that can make people think twice about instigating change; a person who drinks too much may have to change his social circle, for example. Thus people tend to weigh up the perceived benefits, threats and anticipated outcomes of change before they embark on change. Importantly, though, before people enter into change they need to feel that it is within their power to actually change. They need to believe that they possess the will power, strategies, resources and support to be successful. This confidence in the ability to succeed is termed self-efficacy. If people don't believe this, they won't even attempt change. Our job as health promoters is to help people with this decision-making process, increase self-efficacy and facilitate empowerment by providing support and practical help for change. Figure 6.1 shows how an individual may follow the health belief model when weighing up the pros and cons for adopting safe sexual practices in an attempt to lessen his or her risk of becoming HIV positive.

## Brief advice

Another important catalyst for people starting to undertake behaviour change, and one which is important for health professionals to be aware of, is that the public respond to being advised to change their behaviour by someone who is respected and seen as knowledgeable. A systematic review of research studies has shown that brief advice lasting no more than three minutes has been shown to increase a person's chance of quitting smoking by up to 3 per cent (Cochrane Collaboration 2008). This may be seen as a relatively small percentage, but taken on a population level and considering the number of people in day-to-day contact with health professionals it equates to a large number of people for such a quick and easy intervention. Obviously this percentage can be increased by signposting people to specialist services and providing longer, more in-depth consultations. One example of this brief advice or invention technique is the 5As model (ask, advise, assess, assist and arrange). The model encourages health care workers to:

- *Ask* – Raise an issue with their clients, for example, 'Do you smoke?'
- *Advise* – Provide information on the hazards of smoking and advise quitting.
- *Assess* – Assess the client's motivation to change. This could be done by questioning, for example, 'On a scale of 1–10, how motivated are you to quit at the moment?' This stage should also include assessment of the client's pattern of smoking, their previous quit attempts, etc.
- *Assist* – This is the action planning stage in which the health promoter and client work together to set goals and agree on a strategy to achieve these goals. This will include information on the support services resources available to aid the client in their behaviour change. Client confidence with this action plan may be assessed by asking the question, 'On a scale of 1–10, how confident are you of being able to quit?'
- *Arrange* – This stage involves referral or signposting to specialist services, for example a specialist smoking cessation service.

The 5As were devised for use by doctors and other primary care professionals to raise lifestyle issues with their patients, and form the basis of a UK government policy 'Every Contact Counts': 'Every healthcare professional should "make every contact count": use every contact with an individual to maintain or improve their mental and physical health and wellbeing where possible' (NHS Future Forum 2012, p. 11). Health professionals are encouraged to identify five-minute 'windows of opportunity' to discuss lifestyle issues with their clients and follow this model (DH 2010). There are obvious limitations with this model. The limited amount of time health care professionals spend on regular consultations with their clients means it is doubtful whether any purposeful assessment may result. Criticism of the policy includes whether people will feel hounded when attending their doctor, nurse or health visitor for an unrelated topic when the subject of their smoking status, alcohol intake or weight is raised. The fear is that some people will stay away in case they become subjected to this. On the other side of the argument, opportunistic blood pressure checks and chat about lifestyle seems natural and holistic care. However, with the existing pressure on health professionals' time it remains to be seen whether this policy is in fact implemented. A US study into family doctor and nurse use of the brief intervention 5As approach showed little evidence that this was carried out (Dosh *et al.* 2005). Brief intervention does not provide the opportunity for any in-depth assessment of client motivation or matching goals and support to individual circumstances. Nevertheless, health professionals do have a duty to raise lifestyle issues with their patients. Generally, people are well aware themselves of the basic healthy lifestyle messages, so this brief intervention is perhaps best used in signposting people to more specialist health promotion services that can spend more time with patients and provide them with an in-depth assessment of their own individual needs and provide the necessary continuing support for behaviour change.

## The transtheoretical model (stages of change model)

For more in-depth work with clients on behaviour change, Prochaska and DiClemente's (1984) model is a well-recognised and commonly used behavioural change tool. The model begins by assessing a client's motivation to change. Questions are asked of the client such as, 'Have you ever thought that you perhaps needed to cut down your alcohol intake/quit smoking?' It is important that such questions are raised without making a judgement and in a chatty, open manner. The client's reply to exploratory questions allows the health promoter to categorise the client as being in a particular stage of the cycle of change. They may answer that they do not want to change, in which case Prochaska and DiClemente would categorise them as being in the pre-contemplation stage, not interested in changing at the present time. If this is the case, the health promoter's best response would be along the lines of, 'Well, if you do ever get to the stage when you are considering changing, please come and see me, because there is a lot of help we can give you to help you quit'. They may reply that they would like to quit but doubt that they would be successful, or have tried before and failed. They would then be categorised as being in the contemplation phase of the cycle. It is the health promoter's job in this case to build up their confidence, undertake a detailed assessment of their circumstances and habits, and work with them to move them to the next stage of the cycle – the planning stage. In this

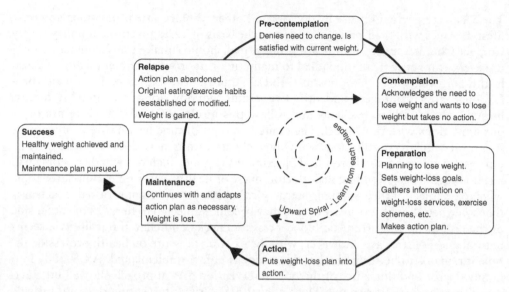

**Figure 6.2** Adaptation of Prochaska and DiClemente's (1983) transtheoretical model to show stages of change for clients undertaking weight loss

stage any previous history of change attempts are explored – What helped? What do they think went wrong? – and goals are set and action plans drawn up. With smoking cessation this will involve setting a quit date and deciding on the use of pharmaceutical products, such as nicotine replacement therapy, bupropion or varenicline, to help with nicotine withdrawal symptoms. The next stage, making changes, is to put the plan into action with the ongoing support of the health promoter. This means regular follow-up appointments and a reassessment of the action plan with changes made as necessary. Hopefully the client will then enter the maintenance phase and adopt the behaviour change long-term, again with the help of follow-up appointments as necessary. Successful long-term behaviour change lasting for six months or more will then mean that they will exit the cycle. However, many people relapse and go on to this stage of the cycle. Relapsing is considered a normal phase of behaviour change, especially for those people who are trying to change for the first time. It is important for the health promoter to convey to the client that relapsing can act as a positive learning experience. It is rare that people succeed first time around with any behaviour change, but lessons will have been learnt that can prove invaluable during the next attempt. The client may wish to take a break and try again another time, and the health promoter needs to leave the door open and encourage to try again at a future date. Figure 6.2 shows an example of using the model to recognise the stages of change in an individual pursuing weight loss.

## Motivational interviewing (MI)

Motivational interviewing is another tried and tested approach in the field of behaviour change. It has proven to be particularly effective when working with the *ambivalent*, pre-contemplative/early contemplative client, where motivation for change appears to be either very low or, at best, 'hanging in the balance', thus holding the client in a position of inertia.

## Background

MI is an empirically supported, testable clinical approach to facilitating constructive conversations about change. It first emerged in 1983 in an article written by its originator, Dr William R. Miller (1983). At that time the prevailing culture consisted of a coercive and confrontational style, intent on inundating people with harsh facts and poor prognosis data as a means of trying to bring about the changes deemed necessary in the best interest of their recovery. Motivational interviewing was presented as an alternative approach and from that point on and since the early 1990s, in partnership with Dr Stephen Rollnick, MI has continued to evolve and develop into an authoritative, strongly evidence-based approach to resolving the common challenges faced by those involved in the field of behaviour change work. Clients can present to professionals at a point in their life or stage of change where they have recognised that there is a problem and have in some way acknowledged that 'something does indeed need to change'. They may have knocked on our door and willingly asked for help. Even so, the health promoter's journey with most clients is likely to encounter some pressure points and obstacles along the way towards the proposed change goal. The challenge is likely to be much greater with clients who are *less* ready, willing and/or able to make changes, for example those who have been sent to services by a third party. This may be a family doctor or a concerned parent or partner, or because a certain set of unexpected circumstances have arisen (e.g. a recent health scare, accident or acute episode, an unplanned pregnancy, an arrest for a drink-driving offence or possession of illegal substances). While for some people such events may serve as a catalyst or prompt for change, others may not be at a stage of recognition and acknowledgement at all; they may even be resentful, offended or angry about the intervention, and could almost certainly be described as averse to, pre-contemplative or ambivalent about behaviour change. This discord or oppositional position can manifest itself in a client's negative body language, poor attendance at services or increased levels of anti-change language, for example utterances such as: 'Yes, but . . .', 'I've tried that before and it didn't work', 'Everyone is just making too big a deal out of this', 'All my friends drink as much as I do and no one is giving them a hard time', 'Well, have *you* ever had this problem?', 'It never did her any harm . . .', and so on. Today research continues to demonstrate that, when met with such client ambivalence, many practitioners will resort to providing clients with what they seem to be 'lacking'; that is, unsolicited advice, information, knowledge, insight or skills associated with the issue in question. This is provided with the well-intentioned aim of using a good argument to 'convince' them to change for their own good, yet often with very limited positive effect. MI offers instead a way of eliciting from people *their own* thoughts, concerns, views and ideas about change, so motivation is *evoked* rather than installed. It builds on the belief that an overly directive practitioner style is counter-productive when ambivalence is observed in the client, and may engender counter change or an oppositional stance from the client. MI conversations can vary in length from very brief – just a few informal minutes – to longer therapeutic sessions of an hour or so. They can take place with individuals or groups from a diverse range of ages and backgrounds and across a broad range of subject areas, homogenous and heterogeneous. The MI practitioner's attitude is always one of warmth, openness and genuine curiosity about the client's dilemma, coupled with a gentle guiding approach to encourage them to move forward. The practitioner aims to cultivate a respectful and collaborative environment within which client receptivity and readiness for change can be skilfully explored and increased. 'It is designed to strengthen an individual's motivation for and movement toward a specific goal by eliciting and exploring the person's own reasons for change within an atmosphere of acceptance and compassion' (Miller and Rollnick 2012, p. 5).

## How does MI work?

MI is a strengths-based approach that utilises a four-process model – (1) engage, (2) focus, (3) evoke, (4) plan – in conjunction with a core set of person-centred micro-skills (OARS) – open questions, affirmations, reflections and summaries. These fundamental components are skilfully woven together and imbued with the qualities of acceptance and compassion (spirit), to *guide* people towards resolving their own change dilemma and to develop commitment to their own change goal. There is a particular focus on the language of change and commitment (change talk) and the practitioner skilfully endeavours to increase the quantity and strength of genuine change talk expressed by the client by mindfully avoiding the traps that encourage defensiveness and counter-change language (the latter of which is shown to decrease the likelihood of change outcomes).

## The four processes

The processes are both sequential and recursive in nature, rather than worked through in rigid stages or phases. They form a semi-structured framework, a sort of compass bearing or reference point for the flow and direction of the MI conversation.

(1) *Engage* – Therapeutic engagement, or a positive practitioner–client relationship, is seen as a necessary precursor to all that follows. The quality of the relationship as rated by the client is a strong predictor of retention and outcome. Engagement is necessary throughout the intervention and not simply at the outset.
(2) *Focus* – Leading naturally from engaging to a spotlight on a particular agenda, i.e. what the person came to talk about, balanced with some things the practitioner may need to raise or cover. This is a collaborative process of clarifying and agreeing the direction of travel and the change hopes/targets/goals for the session(s).
(3) *Evoke* – This is at the heart of MI and involves drawing from the client their own ideas about why and how they might go about making the change. It is the opposite of being expert-led or directive and utilises the client's own wisdom and insight at the core of the intervention.
(4) *Plan* – This is when readiness for change builds to a tipping point and the energy subtly shifts towards the 'how, where and when' of change and away from the 'why' of change. Planning encompasses both the development of an action plan as well as commitment to carrying through with the plan. (A plan without commitment is not a strong indicator of change.)

## *The micro-skills: OARS*

These are the conduit for excellent person-centred communication, as it is through skilful use of these four elements that the entire MI conversation takes place.

- *Open questions* – Used to open up and encourage conversation flow, evoke expression of client's thoughts and insights and minimise short one-word answers where possible. They usually begin, 'How might you . . .', 'Tell me about . . .', 'What are your thoughts on . . .', etc. In general, practitioners tend to rely heavily on questions, and in MI there is much more reliance on the use of reflection (see below). A ratio of one question to two or three reflections is a useful guide for an MI conversation.
- *Affirmations* – Statements of validation or confirmation, usually about strengths, values, qualities, efforts, etc., that the practitioner has noticed in the client and offered to them in the form of a reflective verbal 'gift'. Research shows that effective affirmation leads to an increase in client change talk (see below). Tips for good affirmation include being genuine – don't offer it if you don't mean it – specific rather than general – e.g. 'You have made a big effort not to smoke in the same room as the children' rather than 'You've been trying hard' – and to use it sparingly where it will have most impact (like seasoning in food – it can be overused!).
- *Reflections* – By far the communication skill used most frequently and strategically by the MI practitioner. Reflections can be simple, like sticking closely to the words used by the client, or more complex, where the practitioner aims to be more interpretive by imagining walking in the client's shoes, or by using a range of specific reflection strategies to encourage particular responses, e.g. use of a double-sided reflection to illuminate the ambivalence that is keeping the client stuck. For example, the practitioner may say, 'So, on the one hand you really enjoy cooking and entertaining and holding parties, and on the other you are feeling increasingly unhappy about the way your weight is affecting your confidence in social situations'. A good reflection encourages the client to reach inside and share more of their internal world, like holding a mirror up to their expressed thoughts, which can really help them explore and gain a deeper understanding of their dilemma. Tips for good reflection include trying to avoid the use of lots of sentence stems such as, 'So it sounds like . . .', 'It seems like you may be saying . . .', 'So . . .', ''I think I'm right in hearing you say . . .', etc. It is generally preferable to use less of this type of 'therapy' language and keep the flow more conversational in style. Also, it is not necessary to tag an open question onto the end of every reflection. Try to trust the process and let the reflection resonate with the client.
- *Summaries* – Offered periodically throughout the conversation as a means of providing punctuation and pace, and demonstrating accurate listening to the client. Used strategically to emphasise and possibly link certain relevant themes and to re-emphasise important elements such as client change talk statements. Also used strategically to encourage a gentle forward direction to the conversation and to avoid repetition and 'going around in circles'. Tips for summaries include keeping it simple – less is often more, you do not need to include everything in a summary!

## Information and giving advice in MI

Due to the person-centred nature of the micro-skills (OARS) and the spirit, many practitioners mistakenly interpret MI as an approach that does not allow for the giving of information or advice. This is not the case as MI is both person centred *and* goal oriented. What is important, however, is the when and how of this type of exchange. A useful format – elicit, provide, elicit (E-P-E) – has been developed to help keep the process within MI 'territory' by asking permission to share, and assuming that people have knowledge and insight that should be 'mined' before bringing in any additional information. This style of exchange helps us avoid the expert trap – that is to say, 'I am right and you are wrong'. In action and delivered through use of OARS, it may sound something like the dialogue in the following activity.

### Activity

You are a health visitor discussing childhood immunisations with a mother at a baby clinic. How would you gauge and respond to the mother's anxiety regarding vaccinating her child?

Mother: I don't like the idea of having him vaccinated.

It may be tempting to jump in and provide information about the benefits of vaccination. Instead, like in any nursing intervention, there is first the need to assess. Anxieties, expectations and information the mother already holds need to be elicited.

Health visitor: So tell me what you've heard about the baby immunisation programme. [*First elicit.*]

Mother: It sometimes goes wrong, doesn't it? I mean, you don't know what's in that stuff, or if it will cause more harm than good. It's not natural.

Rather than contradicting the mother, the health visitor seeks to understand and respect her anxieties, affirming her concerns.

Health visitor: You have been really thinking about what's best for your baby, and you want to do the right thing. [*Empathic reflection.*]

Mother: Well, I've read stuff about it causing disabilities in certain children and I don't want to risk that.

Health visitor: Have you got some specific concerns that you'd like to discuss today? [*Reflection.*] Would you like me to go through some of the information about why we encourage immunisation in babies, including some of the potential risks, to see what you think? [*Asking permission to provide information.*]

The health visitor then presents information in a *neutral* fashion, using prefixes such as, 'What the research has shown . . .', 'What other parents have said . . .', etc., rather than, 'I think you should . . .', or, 'What you need to do is . . .'.

Health visitor: What do you make of that? What are your thoughts at this point? [*Final elicit.*]

This final elicit is designed to check out understanding and allows the parent to agree or disagree with the information without it seeming like a personal disagreement, thus maintaining the client–practitioner relationship. It is most important not to pressurise; the client needs time and space to consider. However, providing written information, details of websites, and so on, may be useful to help her with the decision. If the mother is unable to reach a decision at this point, the health visitor can follow this up at a later date.

## The ethos or key principles of MI

### Spirit
A set of values or ethics that serve as a reminder that MI is not simply a box of tools or techniques, 'but a way of being with and for people, the mind-set and heart-set from which one practices MI' (Rollnick and Miller 1995). The following four headings go some way to encompassing the intention of this essential aspect of MI

### Partnership
MI is something that is carried out collaboratively with and for others and not something that is imposed, inflicted or 'done to' them. The practitioner makes every effort to reduce the inevitable power dynamic that exists between 'professional' and 'client' by relating to them as another human being, and by exploring, acknowledging and respecting the expertise they bring from their own life and experiences.

### Acceptance
Sub-divided into four categories: absolute worth, autonomy, accurate empathy and affirmation. In summary,

> taken together, these four person centred conditions convey what we mean by acceptance. One honours each person's *absolute worth* and potential as a human being, recognises and supports the person's irrevocable *autonomy* to choose his or her own way, seeks through *accurate empathy* to understand the other's perspective, and *affirms* the person's strengths and efforts.
>
> (Miller and Rollnick 2012; italics in original)

## Compassion

A genuine desire for the well-being of others, this is not just about being nice and kind but is 'the wish to see others free from suffering' (Dalai Lama 2013). The practitioner actively prioritises the needs and welfare of the client.

## Evocation

The strengths-based approach to eliciting answers and solutions from the client. This is based on the belief that most people have the necessary internal resources to resolve their issues, especially with a little help to draw them forth, rather than on a deficit model that looks for shortcomings, so that these can be corrected or reinstalled from the expert position.

## Change talk

Change talk is perceived in a unique way in motivational interviewing. It refers to the language of change as expressed by the client during the session and is significantly linked to the prediction of outcome. The MI practitioner intentionally seeks to encourage and increase levels of genuine client change talk by utilising all of the aforementioned skills and avoiding traps that may incur the elicitation of sustain talk (language which supports the status quo). Change talk can be considered in two phases: the preparatory phase and the mobilising phase. The first category includes desire, ability, reason and need for change (DARN) and is more prevalent during the earlier stages of change; that is, when ambivalence is still a significant feature of the conversation.

### (1) Preparatory change talk (DARN)

- *Desire* for change, e.g. 'I *wish* I was fit enough to go running with my friend'.
- *Ability* to change, e.g. 'I think I *could* give up smoking if I put my mind to it'.
- *Reason(s)* for change, e.g. 'I want to lose weight to *look good for my wedding* in six months'.
- *Need* for change, e.g. 'With my family history of breast cancer, I really *need* to cut my drinking right down'.

The second phase comes into place as ambivalence is resolving and there is an increase in momentum and volition towards the change goal. It includes commitment, activation and taking steps (CAT). It is important that an MI practitioner can recognise, elicit and respond to change talk as well as differentiate between the categories in order to adjust their response accordingly. Missing the opportunity to shift gear when a client has subtly indicated a nudge towards change can result in a decline in their motivation.

### (2) Mobilising change talk (CAT)

- *Commitment* to change, e.g. 'I *will* start going to the quit smoking group next week', 'I *promise* . . .', 'I *am* definitely going to . . .', etc.

- *Activation* – signs of being ready, willing and able; preparing for change.
- *Taking steps* – evidence and examples of change beginning/happening in current time frame.

Research has shown that when sufficient and appropriately matched attention is given to client DARN language (usually in the form of reflection, affirmation or evocative questioning) a corresponding increase in CAT language is observed, indicating an enhanced likelihood of actual change.

## Key messages

- Health professionals should opportunistically raise the issue of behaviour change with their clients.
- When considering behaviour change, people weigh up the costs and benefits of what the change will mean to them.
- It is important that practitioners are aware of services and techniques that can support clients through behaviour change, and these are discussed with rather than imposed on clients.
- Some clients are able to instigate and maintain behaviour change themselves, others require more support.
- Supporting people who find behaviour change difficult requires in-depth assessment of their ability and motivation to change. This exploratory conversation and relationship-building is key and needs time.
- A person-centred approach that is affirmative of a client's actions is much more likely to be effective than a directive approach, 'being with' clients rather than 'doing to' clients.
- It is important to work with a client's experience, skills and knowledge of themselves and their circumstances to formulate solutions rather than imposing solutions on them.
- Motivational interviewing is a useful series of techniques that can be used to support clients who are ambivalent regarding behaviour change.
- Positive change talk used by the client, especially commitment language, is a strong predictor of actual change.

## References

Cochrane Collaboration (2008) *Physician Advice for Smoking Cessation* (Review). London: Wiley and Sons.

Dalai Lama (2013) *Teachings*. Available online: http://www.dalailama.com/teachings/training-the-mind/verse-2.

DH (Department of Health) (2010) *Healthy Lives, Healthy People: Our strategy for public health in England*. London: Department of Health.

Dosh, S., Holtrop, J., Torres, T., Arnold, A., Bauman, J. and White, L. (2005) 'Changing organizational constructs into functional tools: An assessment of the 5 A's in primary care practices'. *Annals of Family Medicine* 3(Suppl 2): 50–2.

Miller, W.R. (1983) 'Motivational interviewing with problem drinkers'. *Behavioural Psychotherapy* 11: 147–72.

Miller, W.R. and Rollnick, S. (2012) *Motivational Interviewing: Helping people change* (3rd edn). Guilford: Guilford Press.

NHS Future Forum (2012) *The NHS's Role in the Public's Health*. London: Department of Health.

Nutbeam, D. and Harris, E. (2004) *Theory in a Nutshell: A practical guide to health promotion theories*. Sydney, NSW: McGraw-Hill.

Prochaska, J. and DiClemente, C. (1984) *The Transtheoretical Approach: Crossing traditional boundaries of change*. Homewood, IL: Dow Jones-Irwin.

Rollnick, S. and Miller, W.R. (1995) 'What is motivational interviewing?' *Behavioural and Cognitive Psychotherapy* 23: 325–34.

Rosenstock, I.M., Strecher, V.J. and Becker, M.H. (1988) 'Social learning theory and the health belief model'. *Health Education Behavior* 15(2): 175–83.

# 7 Programme planning

*Susan R. Thompson,
Claire Novak and
Kate Thompson*

## Levels of intervention

Public health programmes tend to be categorised in terms of primary, secondary and tertiary prevention programmes. Primary prevention programmes are designed to tackle the determinants or causes of certain conditions in order to prevent that condition from occurring. There are many such interventions in place to do this, and these form much of the focus of the work of health promoters and primary health care professionals. Tackling obesity in order to prevent CVD and diabetes, for instance, or providing free condoms and sexual health advice to reduce the possibility of teenage pregnancy are just two examples. Secondary prevention is work done in order to prevent an existing condition worsening; giving medication or performing coronary angioplasty to patients with angina to stop their condition proceeding to a heart attack is such an example. Tertiary prevention is preventing the complications of an existing condition; for example, people with diabetes are at risk of developing diabetic retinopathy or poor circulation which may lead to leg ulcers and poor healing ability. It is important, therefore, that blood-sugar levels are carefully controlled and diabetics are given regular monitoring appointments to screen for such complications and given advice regarding appropriate self-care so risks may be reduced. Health services engage in all three levels of prevention, but other agencies, such as local authorities, are more able to be involved in primary prevention than secondary or tertiary prevention. However, organisations such as patient groups and voluntary agencies may be involved (certainly in providing information) at all three levels.

Interventions also vary in intrusiveness. Some low-level or potential future health issues are just monitored and no other intervention is proposed. Interventions range from this monitoring, to information provision, incentives and disincentives for individual behaviour change, to restricting or legislating to eliminate a choice seen to directly impact on health. These different levels of interventions are illustrated in the Nuffield Council of Bioethics Ladder of Interventions (2007) (Figure 7.1). The level of intervention proposed is dependent on the number of people affected, the seriousness of the health issue and the cost of it to the economy and health services.

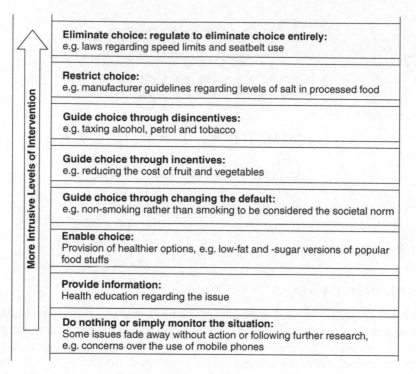

**Figure 7.1** The intervention ladder (Nuffield Council of Ethics 2007)

## Policy-makers

Below is a list of the main public and private bodies who set or contribute to public health policies:

- Government health departments and health ministers. These are strongly influenced by the ethos of the political party in power, which means health policy and direction can suddenly change and policies adopted by one government can be overthrown by the next. A constant 'reform' agenda can be destabilising for health services, and funding can fluctuate depending on government priorities and the wealth of the economy. On close inspection, however, it can be seen that many health and public health policies persist through changes in governments. The policy to reduce health inequalities is one such persistent goal. Language used and rhetoric may alter, with similar policies given new names but remaining largely the same. Health priorities may differ according to political party along with the methods employed to achieve the desired outcomes.
- Health services, regional or local strategic health boards generally implement government priorities, but also have power to make decisions that are seen as responding to the specific needs of their community.
- Local authorities have the potential to set policies to tackle a wide range of health determinants. In England they have been given the power to commission

public health services via local health and well-being boards following joint strategic needs assessments.

- Advisory bodies such as the National Institute for Health and Care Excellence analyse current research and evidence of effectiveness and cost-effectiveness of interventions and advise policy-makers accordingly.
- Professional bodies such as nursing and medical associations gather members' views and lobby for or against changes in policy.
- Single issue groups, for example Action on Smoking for Health (ASH), lobby policy-makers on specific public health issues.
- Independent commissions and inquiries are often commissioned by the government to monitor standards or examine a specific issue and provide reports with the aim of influencing policy. Examples are the Health Care Commission, The King's Fund and the Acheson Inquiry into Inequalities in Health.

## Risk versus benefit analysis

Public health services generally use data regarding known associations or cause and effects to decide on programmes that target certain individuals and communities considered at high risk of developing certain diseases, injuries or social issues. This is seen as a cost-effective use of resources; for example, the individual calculation of CVD risk and the subsequent treatment regimens discussed in Chapter 2. Certain at-risk populations are also targeted; young people truanting from school are at greater risk of developing a drug habit than their more affluent peers (Drug Education Forum 2013), so preventative services may be set up targeted at these individuals and not others. Another benefit of targeting high-risk populations is that both staff and client motivation may be high, as the intervention is seen as relevant to the client group and the benefit versus risk ratio is higher (Davies and Macdowall 2006). Alternatively, an approach that includes the whole of the population may be seen as wasteful, as many of those targeted will not benefit. The Framington coronary heart disease study showed that if all men up to the age of 55 years reduced their cholesterol levels by 10 per cent, one man in 50 would avoid a heart attack, but the remaining 49 would have eaten a healthier diet without actually needing to (Rose 1992). When statistics such as one man in 50 are scaled up to a population level the actual numbers are impressive and significant for governments and health services trying to reduce the cost of such diseases. However, the cost for the individual is high. The risk of a woman contracting HIV from an infected partner during unprotected penile–vaginal intercourse is one in a thousand (CDC 2013), yet the risk is probably perceived to be much higher due to the publicity of the safe-sex message and the profile of HIV in the public's consciousness. Public health is about ensuring the best possible health for the population, but in order to achieve this the risks for the individual are often overemphasised.

## The planning cycle

The first stage of programme planning is to establish a need and hence a rationale for instigating a programme in the first place. As seen in Chapter 4, health needs

Table 7.1 Agencies and actions working together to improve road safety

| | |
|---|---|
| Police | Prosecution of driving offences, speed cameras |
| Highways Agency | Speed bumps, 20 mile/hr zone near schools, pedestrian crossings |
| Education Authority | School bus provision, school crossing patrols |
| Driving Standards Authority | Set standards for driver competence |
| Parent Groups | Organise volunteer walk-to-school schemes |

assessment can take many forms, and when completed the results of needs assessments are used to formulate the strategic plans of organisations that consider policies and programmes to address the needs identified and prioritised. Strategic plans should encompass all agencies who have a responsibility or influence with regard to the issue in question. This 'joined up working' ensures that different aspects of the need are addressed and that all partner organisations work towards common goals. Table 7.1 gives examples of how different agencies may contribute to improving road safety, a primary prevention intervention. Programme planning involves getting together many different agencies, organisations and client groups for discussions, and the logistics of this is difficult in itself. Different agencies have different planning cycles and different priorities for funding and action. It is essential that a consensus is reached and sources of finance are identified and committed by each agency with roles made clear. A crucial point is that commitment comes from executive heads at the top of each organisation; only then will commitment to action and funding result. Difficulties may emerge following a change of management and therefore priorities. This should be guarded against to ensure sustainability. Time scales need to be kept to if at all possible to prevent slippage and the project drifting. There are many planning models, for example Ewles and Simnett (1999) and Nutbeam and Harris (2004), but most have a similar basic format and follow a logical process (see Figures 7.2 and 7.3). Following a recognised model ensures that programmes have a good chance of being effective and all relevant information is taken into account. Good planning focuses on the achievement of agreed outcomes, makes workers prioritise and justify their activities and enables the pursuit and evaluation of an action plan.

## Planning a programme aimed at reducing teenage pregnancy

Suppose it has been decided that there is a need to tackle the level of teenage pregnancy within a particular locality, possibly in response to government policy. First, the level of the issue should be established by accessing epidemiological and demographic information. Statistics regarding teenage pregnancy are collected by maternity services and collated by Public Health Observatories. It is also important to look at the trends over time. Are incidence rates increasing or decreasing? Possibly if they are decreasing

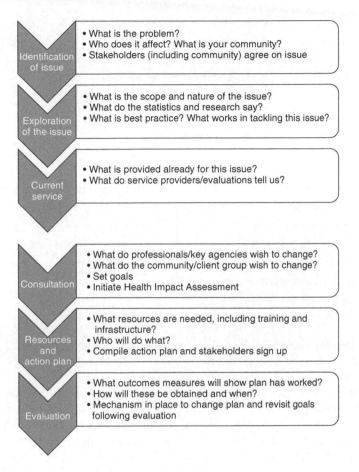

**Identification of issue**
• What is the problem?
• Who does it affect? What is your community?
• Stakeholders (including community) agree on issue

**Exploration of the issue**
• What is the scope and nature of the issue?
• What do the statistics and research say?
• What is best practice? What works in tackling this issue?

**Current service**
• What is provided already for this issue?
• What do service providers/evaluations tell us?

**Consultation**
• What do professionals/key agencies wish to change?
• What do the community/client group wish to change?
• Set goals
• Initiate Health Impact Assessment

**Resources and action plan**
• What resources are needed, including training and infrastructure?
• Who will do what?
• Compile action plan and stakeholders sign up

**Evaluation**
• What outcomes measures will show plan has worked?
• How will these be obtained and when?
• Mechanism in place to change plan and revisit goals following evaluation

**Figure 7.2** Programme planning

at a satisfactory rate there is no need to change the current plan. Key stakeholders, both lay and professional, need to be approached by the organisation taking the lead to ascertain potential involvement in any future project. There should be consultation with local people via community workers or partnership organisations, with the question asked as to whether the rate of teenage pregnancy is a concern to the local population, professionals and voluntary organisations in the area. Ideally, issues to be acted upon should be a priority for local people, not just for health care organisations and the government. A review of the research regarding the determinants or causes of teenage pregnancy should be undertaken, as root causes will need to be addressed if programmes are to be at all effective. Teenage pregnancy is often both a cause and a consequence of social exclusion. Teenage parenthood is more common in deprived areas, amongst those with low educational achievement, young people who are homeless or leaving care and those who are children themselves of teenage parents (Social Exclusion Unit 1999). Next, it is useful to examine evidence from past programmes of

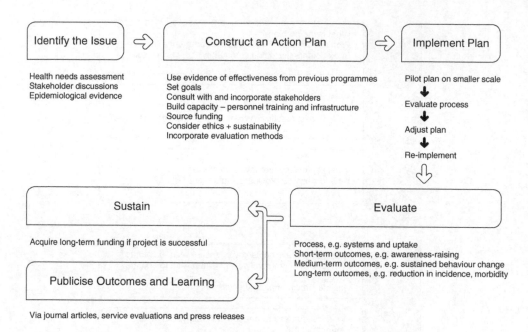

**Figure 7.3** Project planning in health promotion and public health

intervention, locally, nationally and possibly internationally, for similar populations. What seems to have evaluated well and appears to have had some success? In the UK the following fit this criteria: school-based sex education, particularly linked to contraceptive services; community-based education, development and contraceptive services (e.g. operating within youth centres); youth development programmes that focus on personal development, for example programmes that support and teach confidence, self-esteem, negotiation skills, education and vocational development, which may increase contraceptive use and reduce pregnancy rates; and family outreach, including involving the parents of teenagers in information and prevention programmes (NICE 2003). Initiatives should be considered with the logistics, funding and sustainability issues taken into account. Capacity of various stakeholders to contribute should be ascertained and commitment agreed, and consultation on possible action plans should be undertaken with the wider community and local workers. Resources should be identified, including funding required and the cost-effectiveness of interventions considered. Also in need of consideration are what workers – professionals or lay people – are available, what their training needs may be and what infrastructure will be required, such as venues for proposed services. It is useful to garner political and community support for the programme from key community figures and local councillors who will champion the programme, raising awareness and guaranteeing backing for the programmes' initiatives. Health impact assessments need to be carried out (see below) and a pilot planned so initiatives can be tried out and lessons learnt. Evaluation is key and needs to be in place from the very start and during every stage of the programme to establish whether goals have been met. Evaluations are essential if funding is to be secured to sustain the programme into the future and will be required to be rigorous to pass the stringent tests for cost-effectiveness from the various funding bodies supporting the programme. However, due to their nature, health promotion programmes fail to lend themselves to randomised controlled trials, which are considered to be the gold standard by which to prove effectiveness within the medical field. Evaluation should use both quantitative and qualitative methods and consider short-, medium- and long-term outcomes (O'Connor-Fleming *et al.* 2006; Nutbeam 1999; WHO 2001). As most action plans are multifaceted, with many interventions targeted at different aspects of the problem, evaluations need to follow suit. Quantitative statistics regarding teenage pregnancy interventions may consist of recording numbers of young people accessing services as well as over time looking for statistics regarding incidence of teenage conceptions. Qualitative data may be collected regarding service satisfaction and ideas for service development both from clients and staff. Health literacy may be tested, possibly knowledge of the implications of teenage pregnancy in addition to knowledge of service provision pre- and post-conception. As well as reporting on expected outcomes, evaluations may uncover unexpected outcomes, both positive and negative, from the interventions.

## Health impact assessment

Health impact assessment (HIA) has been defined as, 'A combination of procedures, methods or tools by which a policy, programme or project may be judged as to its potential effects on the health of a population' (WHO 1999). Basically, HIA is a consideration of the potential of any policy, programme, project or plan to affect health, both positively and negatively. For example, the world needs to increase its food production due to increasing population numbers, and fertilisers and pesticides are essential tools to do this. However, the health risks associated with these need to be considered to ensure consumers and farmers are not exposed to levels of chemicals that can cause them harm. Many negative results of policy are indirect; for example, opening a factory in a suburban area may be considered to be a good thing for the local economy and jobs, but it will also probably increase traffic congestion and pollution. Increased traffic causes more accidents, increased pollution more respiratory illnesses. Will the jobs actually fit the skill set of local workers, or will workers travel into the area? The combination of the above would make the factory deliver negative outcomes for the local community with little, if any, positives. HIA attempts to predict positive and negative outcomes that may result from proposed policies or programmes to try to mitigate these. To do this it is important that good quality evidence is available to programme planners so predictions will be as accurate as possible. These predictions may be based on experience of similar programmes or policies in similar areas (Kemm 2001). The difficulty is that policies and programmes are complex and diverse and sometimes competing. HIAs seek to weigh up the balance of harm versus benefit, and are essential if policy impacts are to be understood, harm lessened and overall benefits increased. HIA has a broad reach. HIAs are conducted on proposals as diverse as the siting of a new supermarket or global mining consortiums needing to ensure that their industry is seen to be ethical and responsible. HIAs need to be conducted at the early planning stage to enable proposals to be modified in light of their recommendations so health can be safeguarded and enhanced (Birley 2011). As a health promoter you may be directly involved in HIAs either for specific health or non-health projects; for example, you may be involved in consultation with the community to be affected, an essential stage in gathering evidence regarding potential impact. The World Health Organisation provides a website that gives examples of HIAs and suggests tools for policy-makers to use in order to undertake HIAs when planning policies and programmes (WHO 2013).

## Working with communities to plan interventions

A community may be defined as a body of people joined together by a common denominator. This may be living in the same geographical community, having a particular medical condition or social need or other set of circumstances that binds people together. Community profiling, or assessing the needs of a particular community, is an important first step in working with communities. Information gained from questionnaires, focus groups, social networks, voluntary organisations and neighbourhood groups is essential to achieve a picture of the perceived needs of the community in focus. This primary data married with the secondary epidemiological data and evidence gained from local authorities and health and social care services can create a complete picture of that community.

As well as identifying needs, it is important to consider the resources present in the community – its assets, strengths and existing service provision. This is important to establish before planning projects and initiatives. It also prevents profiles from focusing entirely on unmet needs, which can be both distorting and demoralising (Hawtin and Percy-Smith 2007). When considering workers who will deliver different aspects of the programme it is again important to consider the potential or existing skills present in the community in question. This prevents the 'top-down' approach of outside professionals swooping in and 'doing to' communities. Whether it be a neighbourhood community or one connected by a common issue, individuals in that community will possess valuable insight and knowledge of issues that will not be possessed by outsiders. Utilising these skills by the use of peer educators, for example, can give the project credibility within the community and provide personal development opportunities for the workers in question. Evaluation of the use of peer educators to achieve better long-term project outcomes than by using professionals are inconclusive (Harden *et al.* 2001; Tolli 2012). However, it seems instinctive and has been shown to benefit the educators themselves, increasing their health literacy and self-esteem (Asthana and Halliday 2006). Individuals within communities vary in their engagement with each other and their willingness to be involved in the life of their community. This level of community resource is termed 'social capital' and, although a complex and abstract concept, tools have been devised to measure it. Indicators for social capital include the level of trust in a community, engagement in volunteering, voter turnout and membership of community organisations (Social Capital Research 2004). The inference is that the higher the level of social capital in a community, the more public involvement and commitment to projects and the greater chance of successful interventions. Involvement of the community and a comprehensive needs assessment is used to inform the planning of initiatives and projects and are usually a prerequisite for funding applications. However, gaining input and true representation from a local community, client group or service users is often easier said than done. The first step is to gather together a group of interested parties or stakeholders. For a geographical locality this may be local residents, statutory and voluntary local service providers, local businesses and local councillors. For a specific issue this may be service users and carers, statutory and voluntary agencies and academic experts. The steering group needs to set parameters and terms of reference for the group; for example, geographical boundaries, age ranges, clients with certain characteristics, diagnoses, and so on. It is important to have key players on the steering group, those who have valuable knowledge of the politics (with a small 'p') and history of the community and previous efforts at intervention. This hopefully will highlight sensitivities and limit the risk of blundering in and subsequently alienating the target group. Community development workers, local neighbourhood workers or project workers are an essential resource in this regard. Such volunteers or workers hopefully have developed enough local knowledge and trust within the community to have a 'way in' to key influential community figures and therefore access to the wider community. Knowledge of specific local circumstances and power politics involved are essential in order to get people on board and for potential projects to have a chance of success.

Initial aims will be influenced by epidemiological evidence and normative needs as well as potential funding linked to certain issues and evidence from successful projects. It is not feasible to consult on every aspect of community life, especially within a geographical locality, so subjects for action need to be prioritised. It is important to research into the history of interventions to avoid repeating past mistakes. Only when a full picture has been assimilated can effective engagement within the community be planned and enacted. Workers need to bear in mind that those who speak loudest or are the most active and therefore easier to reach may not be truly representative of the community. Effort needs to be expounded in order to access less-high-profile individuals. The scope of community consultation needs to be decided upon and this may largely depend on resources in both collecting and analysing data. One-to-one doorstep surveys may reach the highest proportion of residents but are very labour-intensive. An alternative would be walking through the area at different times of the day and chatting with local people around key issues. Conducting surveys at local events or online surveys are other alternatives. It is important to ask about the positives as well as the negatives, as some communities can feel tarnished by a bad reputation. Once the views of the community have been sought the data needs to be analysed. Qualitative data can be arranged in themes and summarised and presented with typical quotes. Quantitative data may be presented in graphs and charts. Both will form a report with recommendations for actions, which, in turn, requires consultation. It is important that such a report be accessible to the community under focus as well as professional bodies, therefore it is essential that the language is accessible and free from jargon, and it is useful to include a summary. Dissemination needs to be planned through the local media, community groups and forums.

There are many peripheral benefits for individuals who become involved in the identification of needs, action planning and project work. Participating individuals have the potential to increase their personal skills and gain experience that can benefit both themselves and the community long-term. This capacity-building is an essential aspect of community development work (Henderson and Thomas 2002). It is a fact that more affluent and educated communities are often more able to mobilise on issues than deprived communities due to skills already present in those communities (Murphy 2002).

## A case study of community involvement in a public health project: Smoke-free playgrounds in Nottingham City – an example of tobacco control in action

Nottingham City has had a high smoking prevalence rate for some years. The 2012 Citizens Survey asked 2,000 adults to self-report their smoking status, and 31 per cent identified themselves as smokers, which compares to an England average of 20 per cent (ONS 2012), effectively placing Nottingham's prevalence at the level of the rest of the country ten years ago. The Sustainable Community Strategy (One Nottingham 2009) sets an ambitious target of reducing the adult smoking prevalence to 20 per cent by 2020. As part of the Strategic Tobacco Control Strategy for Nottingham, a range of work streams were identified. This example will outline a piece of work looking to the next generation: how can we make smoking history?

### Identifying the issue

The Putting Health at the Heart of Nottingham event in February 2010 brought together around 180 local citizens, including a group of young people, and their respective city councillors and health, community and neighbourhood colleagues. The focus of the day was to look at health issues, in particular smoking and healthy weight, prevalent in each area of the city and identify what local initiatives could make a difference. The day consisted of workshops in the morning, with each of the nine areas of the city compiling a list of priority actions, followed by a full council debate, during which the outcomes from the morning were discussed. There was an emotive debate on smoking, which included a memorable quote from a parent making reference to smoking in children's playgrounds: 'I don't want my child playing in a giant ashtray.' There is evidence of widespread support amongst smokers and non-smokers for the prohibition of smoking in children's outdoor play areas (Royal College of Physicians 2010).

As part of the full council debate, councillors were asked to support a motion recognising that smoking and healthy weight are cross-party, long-term, strategic priorities for Nottingham. They also considered how effective ideas from the morning session could be in reducing the significant gap in life expectancy between different communities in the city and how they could be implemented. There was unanimous cross-party support for the motion, and councillors also pledged to consider all of the outcomes from the earlier workshops for incorporation into its Sustainable Community Strategy. They committed to establishing a working group involving key councillors and colleagues to consider issues raised from the debate and suggestions made from the workshops. It was agreed that the working group would report directly to the Health and Adult Social Care Select Committee.

A priority action for the working group was to facilitate the introduction of smoke-free children's playgrounds and school gates. There is little substantive evidence regarding any significant health risks around outdoor exposure to second-hand smoke, rather the thrust of the action was about de-normalising smoking. Some more deprived areas of the city have significantly higher rates of smoking, and this approach sought to break the intergenerational cycle. The aim was to use a whole community approach to create a new social norm of a smoke-free Nottingham City.

## Constructing an action plan

The working group brought together Nottingham City Council portfolio holders for health, children and young people, the head of service for parks and open spaces, NHS and tobacco control colleagues. The group reported directly to the Health and Adult Social Care Select Committee, which ensured that it retained political support, and the actions continued to be a priority. A competition was held across Nottingham City primary schools to design the artwork for the smoke-free signage to be used on school gates and playgrounds. Teaching colleagues were provided with a brief that emphasised artwork should focus on children having the opportunity to play in smoke-free environments. The winning artwork would be used at over 90 primary school gates and in 70 council-run playgrounds. In part to maintain political engagement, local councillors helped to choose prize winners. The project also linked in with the Smoke-Free Homes project, a local NHS-funded initiative aiming to raise awareness of the health risks of second-hand smoke and encouraging parents and carers to pledge to make their homes smoke-free.

## Implementing the action plan

A press release was prepared to launch the initiative that focused on three main areas: preventing uptake of smoking by young people, second-hand smoke and litter. It is estimated that smoking-related litter costs the UK £342 million per annum (Nash and Featherstone 2010). In common with many large cities, Nottingham is keen to improve its image and minimise clean-up costs. There is also evidence that discarded cigarette butts pose a choking hazard to children and are toxic if eaten (Navotony *et al.* 2011). The press release message was one from children, not adults, and purposefully did not include a 'quitting' message. The communications team at the local authority were prepared for a reactionary response from local press and radio, along the lines of 'Is this just the "nanny state"?' However, in the event there was overwhelming support from the media around the issue of taking smoking out of sight of children. It was made clear that the issue was not enforceable, but was dependent on the goodwill of Nottingham citizens.

A last-minute glitch occurred with the signage just before the launch. Working in a local authority environment often necessitates the need to adapt work plans and priorities. In this instance, senior politicians required alcohol and dogs to be added to the artwork. So for example, signs read, 'Please keep this playground dog-, alcohol- and smoke-free'. There was concern that this would dilute the message; however, the media picked up and concentrated primarily on the smoke-free element. The launch was at a large, recently renovated, council-run playground and involved prize winners, parents, schools, councillors and colleagues. There was local and national press and TV and radio coverage, and the communications team reported that it generated more media interest than any other story they had worked on. A highlight was *BBC East Midlands Today* reporter Jo Healey reporting live from the event. She was surrounded by a sea of children and was able to raise the issue that 50 children are admitted to hospital due to second-hand smoke every year in Nottingham.

## Evaluation

The results of the evaluation of the project were not available at the time of press, but methods include a survey of local community protection officers (to ascertain their perceptions and numbers of littering fixed-penalty notices issued), sites monitored by parks staff for litter levels, and a survey amongst parents, carers and children to determine attitudinal and behavioural change. Current anecdotal evidence from the local Smoke-Free Homes project suggests a slow cultural shift towards it being unacceptable to smoke around children.

## Publication of outcomes and learning

There has been demand via regional networks to learn from Nottingham's experience and there are plans to disseminate learning more widely once the evaluation is fully completed. For the future there is an intention to train parks staff to give very brief advice messages around smoking. There is also considerable interest to extend the project to include sports clubs, sports venues and all outdoor events.

## Key messages

- Public health programmes may be primary, secondary or tertiary, but health promoters tend to concentrate on primary prevention.
- Programmes are set up usually in response to policies drawn up by national and local governments and health services as a result of health needs assessment.
- Programme planning should bring together agencies and organisations and client groups who are connected with the issue in question.
- Use of a planning model is recommended and can greatly aid the planning process.
- Programmes should undertake health impact assessments of proposed initiatives to ensure programmes will result in positive rather than negative outcomes for the community in question.

## References

Asthana, S. and Halliday, J. (2006) *What Works in Tackling Health Inequalities?* Bristol: The Policy Press
Birley, M. (2011) *Health Impact Assessments: Principles and practice.* Abingdon: Earthscan.

CDC (Centre for Disease Control and Prevention) (2013) Website: http://www.cdc.gov/.

Davies, M. and Macdowall, W. (2006) *Health Promotion Theory*. Maidenhead: Open University Press.

Drug Education Forum (2013) Available online: http://www.drugeducationforum.com/index.cfm?PageID=8.

Ewles, L. and Simnett, I. (1999) *Promoting Health: A practical guide* (4th edn). London: Bailliere Tindall.

Harden, A., Oakley, A. and Olive, S. (2001) 'Peer-delivered health promotion for young people: A systematic review of different study designs'. *Health Education Journal* 60: 339–53.

Hawtin, M. and Percy-Smith, J. (2007) *Community Profiling: A practical guide*. Maidenhead: Open University Press.

Henderson, P. and Thomas, N. (2002) *Skills in Neighbourhood Work* (3rd edn). London: Routledge.

Kemm, J. (2001) 'Health impact assessment: A tool for healthy public policy'. *Health Promotion International* 16(1): 79–85.

Murphy, M. (2002) 'Social partnership: Is it the "only game in town?"' *Community Development Journal* 37(1): 80–90.

Nash, R. and Featherstone, H. (2010) 'Cough up: Balancing tobacco income and costs in society'. *Policy Exchange*.

Navotony, T.E., Hardin, S.N., Hovda, L.K., Novotony, D.J., Mc'Lean, M.K. and Khan, S. (2011) 'Tobacco and cigarette butt consumption in humans and animals'. *Tobacco Control* (Suppl 1): 17–20.

NICE (National Institute for Clinical Excellence) (2003) *Teenage Pregnancy and Parenthood: A review of reviews*. NHS Health Development Agency. Available online: http://www.nice.org.uk/niceMedia/documents/teenpreg_evidence_briefing_summary.pdf.

Nuffield Council of Bioethics (2007) *Public Health Ethical Issues, Executive Summary*. Cambridge: Cambridge Publishers, p. xix.

Nutbeam, D. (1999) 'The challenge to provide "evidence" in health promotion'. *Health Promotion International* 14(2): 99–101.

Nutbeam, D. and Harris, E. (2004) *Theory in a Nutshell: A practical guide to health promotion theories*. Sydney: McGraw-Hill.

O'Connor-Fleming, M.L., Parker, E.A., Higgins, H.C. and Gould, T. (2006) 'A framework for evaluating health promotion programs'. *Health Promotion Journal of Australia* 17(1): 61–6.

One Nottingham (2009) *The Nottingham Plan to 2020 Priority Implementation Plans*. Available online: http://www.nottinghamcity.gov.uk/onenottingham/CHttpHandler.ashx?id=18650&p=0.

ONS (Office for National Statistics) (2012) *Integrated Household Survey 2011/12*.

Rose, G. (1992) *The Strategy of Preventive Medicine*. Oxford: Oxford University Press.

Royal College of Physicians (2010) *Passive Smoking and Children: A report by the Tobacco Advisory Group of the Royal College of Physicians*. London: Royal College of Physicians.

Social Capital Research (2004) *Measurement of Social Capital*. Available online: http://www.socialcapitalresearch.com/literature/operationalisation/measurement.htm.

Social Exclusion Unit (1999) *Teenage Pregnancy Report*. London: Stationery Office.

Tolli, M.V. (2012) 'Effectiveness of peer education interventions for HIV prevention, adolescent pregnancy prevention and sexual health promotion for young people: A systematic review of European studies'. *Health Education Research* 27(5): 904–13.

WHO (World Health Organisation) (1999) *Definition of HIA*. Available online: http://www.who.int/hia/about/defin/en/index.html.

WHO (World Health Organisation) (2001) *Evaluation in Health Promotion: Principles and perspectives*. Available online: http://www.euro.who.int/__data/assets/pdf_file/0007/108934/E73455.pdf.

WHO (World Health Organisation) (2013) *Health Impact Assessment*. Available online: http://www.who.int/hia/en/.

# 8 The same or different?

## Health promotion in ethnically diverse communities

### *Vanessa McFarlane*

This chapter will look at how health promotion work can be delivered to meet the needs of ever-changing, diverse population groups. It will aim to identify target communities and discuss how health inequalities impact on these groups. It will also consider whether ethnic minority health requires the provision of separate, specific services for our ethnically diverse population or if this may in fact widen the gap between ethnic minorities and the general population. It will also examine evidence of best practice and the resources available to health promoters working with such client groups.

## Minority ethnic identities within the UK

The ethnic mix of the UK population has changed incredibly over the past 60–70 years and the terms to describe non-white groups have also undergone many changes within this period. Once referred to as 'coloureds' (or worse), the term 'ethnic minorities' would often refer to people of African Caribbean origin or those from the Indian subcontinent. This was replaced by 'black and minority ethnic (BME)', which aimed to be more inclusive of those who didn't fall into the African Caribbean or Asian categories, and more recently the acronym BAMER (black, Asian minority ethnic and refugee) is being applied with an aim to be more inclusive in a changing environment. The name change reflects the challenge of trying to include all those from ethnic minority groups under one banner, which is a near on impossible task. This chapter will use the term BME, which includes refugee and asylum-seeking communities. An individual's ethnicity is subjective. People have their own view of who they are based on where they were born, where their parents or family were born, the culture they fit into, the religion they adhere to, and so on, and this is much more complex and makes the job of fitting into an ethnic category difficult. 'Ethnicity is a socially constructed concept including elements of culture, place of birth and skin colour, and there is no adequate measure of it' (PHE 2013).

## UK demographics

Over 80 per cent of the population of England and Wales classify themselves as white British (UK Government 2012), so those from other ethnic groups are still very much the minority within UK society. The 2011 census shows that in England and Wales, Asian/Asian-British and black African/Caribbean/black British are the second and third largest populations respectively after white British (UK Government 2012). These communities were the first wave of immigrants to come to the UK from the late 1940s onwards. The push factors in countries of origin included poverty, unemployment, and political unrest in the case of Kenyan and Ugandan Asians. The pull factor was the need for workers to rebuild a war-torn nation, so the UK government invited people from Commonwealth countries and British-owned territories to come to the 'motherland' and work. Many people came with the intention to work hard, send money home and eventually return to their country of origin. However, once in the UK the realities were very different, and the newcomers were only able to get low-paid, menial jobs, along with substandard housing. This meant it was very difficult to return 'home'. These communities are now established and over the years the pattern of immigration has changed. Forty-one per cent of migrants to the UK in 2011 were foreign students entering temporarily for a course of study, with economic migrants (those seeking work) accounting for 32 per cent of the total (The Migration Observatory 2013). Although recent expansion of the European Union has resulted in Eastern Europeans migrating to the UK, 55 per cent of current migrants to the UK are from outside the EU. Wars and human rights violations have meant an increase in people seeking asylum, having been displaced from their home nation. Nevertheless, despite the publicity, asylum seekers only account for a third of 1 per cent of the UK population (UNHCR 2013). The main countries of origin of asylum seekers to the UK are Pakistan, Iran, Sri Lanka and Nigeria (UNHCR 2013). Recent UK government attempts to limit immigration to the UK by increasing restrictions and strengthening border control are the cause of much debate, but nevertheless every year more people enter the UK than leave it. In 2011 this amounted to 215,000 people (The Migration Observatory 2013). Researchers at the University of Leeds (2013) in the UK have estimated that by 2051 the UK's population will be significantly larger and more diverse than at present and may rise to 20 per cent of the total UK population. They project that the population will rise to 78 million, that the white British, white Irish and black Caribbean groups will experience the slowest growth, while white Other, and Other Ethnic groups will experience the largest growth. It is also predicted that, in common with previous trends, ethnic minorities will gradually move out of inner city areas and integrate more widely within the general population and live in more affluent areas (University of Leeds 2013). However, percentages of ethnic communities are not equally distributed throughout the UK; London has the most diverse community and Wales the least (UK Government 2012). Despite this, in the majority of our major cities diversity is increasing. In recent years new immigrants coming to the UK seeking asylum have been dispersed to areas of England where traditionally there have been very few, if any, people from a different ethnicity; for example, Newcastle saw their BME community grow by 60 per cent to nearly 6.9 per cent of the total population, an increase from 4.1 per cent in 1991 (Newcastle

Joint Strategic Needs Assessment 2013). Both the increase in diverse populations and the greater integration have significant ramifications for the provision of health services. Larger numbers will require increased resources and also the scattering of communities means that neighbourhood services situated in specific ethnic areas (a common current approach to provision) will no longer reach all of those in need. This all presents challenges in the way the health of the nation is addressed. As the population changes, so do the needs of those communities. The health service has to be flexible, understanding, innovative and fair in the way it deals with these new challenges in order to improve the health of all its people.

## Health inequality and ethnicity

There has long been an acknowledgement of the health inequalities experienced by the BME communities in the UK. In 1992 the government's white paper *Health of the Nation* identified key areas where health inequalities disproportionately affect people from BME communities. An example of this was in the area of cancer where it was recognized that in 'terms of screening, treatment and palliative cancer services are not always accessible and sensitive to the needs of this section of the population' (DH 1992). More recently the Marmot Review, *Fair Society, Healthy Lives* (Marmot 2010), strongly documents the impact that socio-economic factors have on health which is compounded by the possession of protected equality characteristics such as race, disability, gender and sexual orientation to name but a few. BME communities tend to hold lower socio-economic positions in society and live in more deprived situations. This is particularly true for those newer communities such as refugees, asylum seekers and migrant workers. The Marmot Review states there are gaps of up to 7 years in life expectancy between the richest and poorest neighbourhoods (Marmot 2010). The more established communities such as the African-Caribbean and Asian communities remain deprived despite being in this country for 70 years in some cases. There has been more movement towards affluence and as new generations are born, this is predicted to increase; however, key health issues persistently disproportionately affect BME communities.

## Refugees and asylum seekers

Kinsi Clarke (Into The Mainstream Project Nottingham) states that in the case of new communities such as refugees and asylum seekers there are issues that are more acute. The language barrier is probably one of the biggest issues and although health services have access to interpreting services this may vary across the country. The interpreting services that can be used over the phone are often perceived as being expensive and inconvenient, which results in a reluctance to use them. Amdani Juma, director of African Initiative for Social Development, states that new entrants also experience a culture shock and a lack of knowledge regarding services available to them. The concept of preventative care such as health promotion can be an unknown concept for many migrants, leaving them with confusion as to the roles played by various professionals within the UK health services. Amdani states that due to a change in lifestyle, people are now suffering with illnesses that they would not have at home, which means health promotion messages have to be culturally appropriate and the message kept simple and easy to understand. In many nations antenatal care is not available and pregnant women only present to health services when they are ready to deliver. Studies show that pregnant asylum seekers are seven times more likely to develop complications relating to pregnancy and birth and three times more likely to die than the general population (RCOG 2004). Primary care and family doctors are also less evident in developing nations where health services are more reliant on secondary care, which again in the UK may result in inappropriate presentation at hospital emergency departments. The situation is further compounded by misunderstanding regarding eligibility for free health care. Those with refugee status and asylum seekers pursuing an application for refugee status are eligible for free NHS care, whereas failed asylum seekers are not (DH 2012). It is also important to appreciate the physical and emotional journey undertaken by refugees and asylum seekers that may have lasted many months or even years. During this journey they may have experienced many traumatic events, including rape, torture and loss of family, which have significant effects on their psychological and physical health. Other common physical health problems suffered by asylum seekers are infectious diseases due to poor immunisation programmes within their home countries, sexually transmitted diseases and poor uptake of contraceptive services and chronic disease (FPH 2008).

## Specific health issues affecting BME communities

### Cardiovascular disease (CVD)

CVD, which includes heart disease, stroke and other diseases of the heart and circulation, is the leading cause of death each year in the UK. Contributing factors are smoking, obesity and high blood pressure (ONS 2011). The British Heart Foundation (2013a) states that 'cardiovascular disease (CVD) can affect different ethnic groups in different ways.' For those people born in South Asia but dying in England and Wales, CVD accounts for almost a quarter of all deaths (BHF 2013a).

Rates of smoking are high among Indian and Bangladeshi men, although rates of binge drinking are lower than the national average in ethnic minority groups. The BHF has stated that simple measurements of obesity cannot accurately measure obesity in ethnic minority groups as fat is stored differently (BHF 2013a).

## Diabetes

The prevalence of diabetes is higher among some BME groups such as Indian, Caribbean, Pakistani and Bangladeshi communities. Global studies on ethnicity and the rising incidence of diabetes tells us that ethnicity can increase or decrease the risk of developing diabetes. Type 2 diabetes, which is most common globally, is up to six times more likely in people of South Asian descent and up to three times more likely in African and African-Caribbean people (Diabetes UK 2010). Studies globally have found that diabetes affects different ethnic groups in different ways. Like CVD, it has a strong association with obesity and links with deprivation due to lower levels of physical activity, poorer diet and poor blood pressure control, and CVD is a major cause of death and disability for people with diabetes.

## Hypertension

Hypertension is a major risk factor for CVD. In the UK, hypertension has been found to be higher in the African, African Caribbean and South Asian populations (defined as people originating from the Indian subcontinent and East Africa). However, for African Caribbean and African populations, stroke and end stage renal failure are more common, while coronary artery disease is more common among South Asians. It is possible that blood pressure (BP) regulation differs between ethnic groups, causing higher BP levels among African Caribbean and South Asian populations, although more research is needed in this field (He *et al.* 1999; Lane and Lip 2001). Hypertension is also strongly associated with lifestyle factors such as obesity, excess dietary salt and smoking. These factors are more prevalent in deprived ethnic communities and the combination of regulatory factors in the body and lifestyle may be the causes of the high rates of hypertension in these groups. Health promotion regarding lifestyle change is therefore a fundamental need to control blood pressure and prevent it leading to CVD.

## Cancer

BME communities tend to have cancer diagnosed later than the general population, which in turn leads to poorer chance of long-term survival (Cancer Equality UK 2013). This is particularly evident in the case of prostate cancer in black men. Prostate cancer is the most common cancer in men in the UK after lung cancer. Black African Caribbean men have approximately a threefold risk of developing prostate cancer at a younger age, and the death rate from prostate cancer is 30 per cent higher in black men compared to their white peers (Thompson 2013). This shows clear health inequality. Cancer Equality UK and BME cancer communities provide advice and resources for health promoters to help them raise awareness of cancer risks within BME communities.

## Mental health

Evidence shows that there is an over-representation of black African, black Caribbean and other black groups in mental health settings (CHAI 2005), and some studies show that African-Caribbeans are between two and eight times more likely to be diagnosed with schizophrenia than the white population (Harrison 2002). African-Caribbeans are also more likely to enter mental health settings via the court system and to be detained under the Mental Health Act than other UK population groups (Mental Health Foundation 2013). BME people are more likely than the general population to be placed in secure mental health settings and have a disproportionately negative experience within these settings. They are more likely to experience a poor outcome from treatment and to disengage from mainstream mental health services, leading to social exclusion and deterioration in their mental health. It is suggested that traditional mental health services are poor at understanding or providing services for non-white communities (Mental Health Foundation 2013).

It is also important to note that non-black ethnic groups also seem to be dispropor- tionately at risk from mental health issues. Researchers have pointed out that the Irish have above-average rates of mental illness, and those born in Ireland but living in the UK had the highest rate of suicide of any ethnic group living in the UK (Fitzpatrick 2005; Mental Health Foundation 2013). This may point to future issues regarding the growing Eastern European population of the UK as deprivation, displacement and cultural issues point to the development of mental health problems.

## Human immunodeficiency virus (HIV)

Black and multi-ethnic communities in the UK are the most severely affected by HIV infection. In 2005, two-thirds of new diagnoses of HIV were among BME groups, with 83 per cent in black African individuals, 6 per cent amongst black Caribbeans and 2.1 per cent amongst South Asian communities (HPA 2005). In 2011 there were 25,331 black Africans living with HIV and accessing care and treatment. This figure has under- gone a fourfold increase in nine years (NAT 2013). It is estimated that approximately 23 per cent of this population remain undiagnosed, and sexually active black Africans are recommended to have yearly HIV tests (NAT 2013). There is an issue with late diagnosis within this group due to a variety of issues such as fear of stigma, denial of exposure to HIV or fear of repatriation if they are asylum seekers. These groups tend to be in the most deprived and vulnerable situation. Health inequalities are marked in this particular area.

## Addressing health inequalities in BME communities

The 2010 Equality Act (UK Government 2010) simplified legislation by encompass- ing all aspects of discrimination law under one act. The NHS is obliged by this law to promote equality across all its activities and service provision. It is important that the NHS is responsive to individual needs and should aim to take account of varying lifestyles, faiths and cultural differences. The NHS already has clear values and prin- ciples about equality and fairness, as set out in the NHS Constitution (2012). These principles involve ensuring that individual patient needs are central to care and pro- viding a comprehensive service for all, therefore no one should be excluded based on any protected characteristic, including ethnic group, culture and religion. In the new world order of commissioning and providers services 'there are legal duties requiring the NHS Commissioning Board and clinical commissioning groups to have regard to the need to reduce inequalities in access to health services and the outcomes achieved for patients' (NHS Handbook 2013, p. 16).

The health promoter plays an essential part in striving to reduce health inequalities, and five key principles have been identified for adapting behavioural interventions for minority ethnic communities which are:

- Use community resources to publicise the intervention and increase accessibility
- Identify and address barriers to access and participation
- Develop communication strategies which are sensitive to language use and information requirements
- Work with cultural or religious values that either promote or hinder attitudinal and behavioural change
- Accommodate varying degrees of cultural identification.

(Netto *et al.* 2010)

These principles now form the basis of NICE guidance.

## Specific services for BME communities

There is ongoing debate regarding whether it is effective and necessary to provide separate services for BME communities. These services are staffed by people from similar cultural or religious backgrounds to the target population. They speak the same languages and understand the barriers to health care experienced by the group that they serve. There are many examples of services, predominantly in the voluntary sector, that are culturally specific and have been very successful. The NAZ Project London (NPL) provides sexual health services and HIV support to BME communities and is the longest and largest established BME charity in the UK. It offers services to the wide and diverse BME communities in London and does this successfully. There are many BME-specific services in the city and their success may be the familiarity of this model and the anonymity people can find in a big city, which is particularly beneficial with an issue such as sexual health and HIV. However, there is evidence that service users return to the service regularly and therefore become known to staff who provide the right level of confidentiality and service to ensure the trust of their client group.

Another example of culturally specific services are services set up for sickle cell and thalassaemia, conditions which only affect African, Caribbean and Asian communities. These services are therefore culturally relevant for their clients and provide important support. Nottingham has had a successful sickle cell service for over 30 years and continues to provide a service to the African, Caribbean and Asian communities. Perhaps in order to address health inequalities amongst BME communities there is a need for specific services for many other health issues, including CVD and diabetes, which, as has been seen, disproportionately affect BME communities, but would this be cost-effective or even work? Lisa Robinson, director of Bright Ideas Nottingham, a community engagement and involvement organisation, believes the key lies in culturally competent services. Lisa feels frustration at statutory services that do not meet the needs of the BME community and often cause a division between BME communities and wider populations. Lisa feels strongly that with the new commissioning system BME provision has lost out. This seems to be particularly noticeable in mental health service provision where BME-specific services that were providing an essential service to the community have been decommissioned.

Lisa and honorary professor Suman Fernando, who lobbies for anti-racist practice in mental health, believe that there is a political move to take BME issues off the agenda. Dr Fernando claims in a *Guardian* article that 'under the coalition government there is a "huge" risk of race falling under the radar altogether' (*The Guardian* 2012). He sees the upheaval of NHS reforms sidelining the vital issue around race and mental health provision. Bright Ideas has seen a tenfold increase in requests to help local services who are struggling to engage BME communities due to their lack of experience, networks and buy-in from the community. There seems to be a lack of willingness by mainstream services to invest in training or buying in advice or expertise to enable them to provide a culturally competent service. This may be due to lack of acknowledgement of the need to be culturally competent or due to budgetary constraints. Lisa does see a need for BME-specific services where need is not met and patients/clients want that service. The service has to be effective, competent and accountable. A good example of this is BME Cancer Communities (2013), founded by Rose Thompson as a response to the unmet needs of BME communities in regard to cancer. Choice is also key. People will vote with their feet, showing expressed need, so mainstream and BME services do need to work together to create culturally competent services.

Dr Chris Udenze, a Nottingham GP, feels that in some areas of health having a culturally specific service is beneficial, and this has been seen in the case of sickle cell and substance misuse. However, the main issue is that staff are culturally sensitive. Dr Udenze's experience with substance misuse patients is that it is a personal issue that is stigmatized and carries racial stereotypes. He also discusses the 'spiritual' aspect involved for those who may have had near-death experiences. It may be more helpful having a worker who has a level of empathy with the client who has experienced this, but alternatively the issue may be too personal and it may be preferable for clients to work with someone who is far removed from their own cultural background. Dr Udenze's opinion is that a service should represent cultural diversity in its staff make-up. The goal should be that all services provide a culturally sensitive and equitable service to all, so everyone can access that service and be treated according to their varying needs the same but different. Amdani Juma, the director of the African Institute for Social Development, feels that building trust is key and that if staff, whatever their ethnicity, maintain a confidential service and show empathy and understanding, talking to someone from the same or different cultural or religious background about sensitive issues should not be a problem.

## BME project case studies

### *Awaredressers Nottingham*

Awaredressers Nottingham is a grass roots outreach community sexual health promotion project. Started ten years ago as a small pilot inspired by a larger project in London, the basic premise of the project is to provide free condoms to the African and Caribbean communities in Nottingham via barbers, hairdressers and other community venues such as studios and community centres. The project is managed by a health promotion specialist and has 22 barbers and hairdressers on board. It has been funded by various sources, but the past four years of funding has come directly from the NHS. The project has taken time to become established and gain the trust of the communities it provides for. Importantly, it has involved participants in decisions about the project, taking ideas and suggestion forward and using them in the project to encourage a sense of ownership. Monitoring has shown that the project reaches both men and women with age ranges from 16 to 50+. The project's main client group is African and Caribbean men between 20 and 30. The project has enabled other health promotion activities such as on-the-spot screening for STIs and visual information to increase awareness about HIV and sexual health services in Nottingham. This project provides qualitative evidence that it works. Year-on-year there has been an increase in condom uptake, which amounted to over 70,000 in 2012–13. Snapshot evaluation shows that clients think the project is a good way to promote sexual health in the BME communities, and condoms are provided in a space that is accessible and comfortable. This is an example of a culturally specific project that aims to fill a gap where there can be barriers to using mainstream services, either because people are not familiar with them or feel they are not appropriate for them, or because services have restricted opening times.

## Bright Ideas Nottingham

Bright Ideas, an organisation specialising in increasing engagement by BME communities, has been commissioned by the British Heart Foundation (BHF 2013b) to help it work with BME communities more effectively. The partnership has produced a series of initiatives, including those detailed below:

- *Reggaerobics* – a program aimed at increasing physical activity within the community. Classes are free and held at an easily accessible local venue. It has been very successful and classes have seen up to 64 people attend.
- *Local radio* – Bright Ideas joined up with local urban radio station 97.5 Kemet FM to deliver a series of adverts to raise awareness about salt reduction, smoking cessation, physical activity and healthy eating.
- *Come Nyam with Me* – a different take on the TV series *Come Dine with Me*, but coming from a Caribbean point of view. Bright Ideas engaged local restaurants to run cook and eat sessions where traditional dishes are made from the African-Caribbean recipe book developed by the BHF. The focus was on reducing salt and fat and educating people on the nutritional value of food. The BHF distributed thousands of recipe books to support this work.
- *'Patty Dumplin'* – Bright Ideas worked with a local artist Lisa Jackson of Mon0Lisa Productions to develop this 60+ Caribbean female fictional character who is not afraid to tell it like it is when it comes to healthier lifestyles. Patty delivers radio ads and attends events to encourage audience participation.

## Dr Chris Udenze GP (NDU Surgery, Nottingham)

Dr Udenze demonstrates good practice through his one-to-one work. He believes in focusing on an individual's particular needs, not just their diagnosis and medical treatment. The key is to build up trust and confidence by asking questions to build up a comprehensive picture of that individual and then tailor health promotion to that person. There is much debate regarding the lack of time for GP consultations, but

Dr Udenze finds that giving people time to talk does not result in long consultations. If not rushed but made to feel comfortable and encouraged to talk about what their worries and symptoms are, generally people tend to get to the point. He does state that some groups such as refugee and asylum seekers need more time due to the major social issues at play such as housing, legal issues and psychological issues as well as their physical health issues. Dr Udenze encourages patients to bring a list with them to their consultation that they can work through together. In Dr Udenze's experience it is better to work with patients in this way rather than them access A&E inappropriately. He states, 'It's not worth making ten appointments for ten different problems, so make a list so you don't forget anything; it might be one thing causing all ten problems'. Dr Udenze uses motivational interviewing techniques where appropriate; for example, when helping patients with substance misuse problems. Dr Udenze advocates the need for health care services to exhibit high levels of compassion and care. He believes that to improve the health of BME communities the key is communication. It is essential that consultations are comfortable and accepting in order to gain a patient's trust and cooperation.

## Into the Mainstream (ItM)

Into the Mainstream demonstrates a good model of practice when working with refugee and asylum seekers (R&AS), not just because it is solely set up to support R&AS to access health services, but also because it is strategically placed within an organisation that meets the needs of this patient group in a holistic manner by offering a wide range of services under one roof. The project developed from a joint strategic needs assessment (JSNA) between Nottingham City and Nottingham PCT concerning the health needs of R&AS in Nottingham. The findings showed poor access to health services by R&AS communities, which resulted in this project, the main aim of which is to integrate new arrivals to Nottingham into the health system. People arriving in the city are offered a one-to-one consultation. They are then, most importantly, registered with a GP, often accompanied by a project worker. The project then supports them to access other health services that may be needed, such as maternity services, health visitors, dentists, mental health services, sexual health/HIV services and, occasionally, female genital mutilation (FGM) services. The project works both with NHS staff through awareness-raising training and one-to-one contacts/meetings and with patients. This involves explaining to patients how the NHS works while equally informing staff of issues around access and eligibility to health care. As an example, Kinsi Clarke, a senior health project worker, recently spent over three hours at a surgery trying to register a heavily pregnant woman, as staff did not understand who they could or could not register or what documentation was actually required. In another situation practice staff were of the misguided opinion that a woman could not see a midwife without being registered with a GP first. Training has been offered to GP surgeries by the ItM project, but uptake has been low and there is clearly a need for awareness to be raised so clients from R&AS communities have fair and equal access to health services. The project is currently funded for another three years and currently works with two part-time staff (equivalent to 1.5 full-time equivalent posts), which, given the rising client numbers and increasing difficulties to accessing primary services, is not sufficient. But the important point is that this project exists, and without it many people would fall through the net and have no access to health services in Nottingham.

### African Institute for Social Development (AISD)

AISD 'is a volunteer African-led community organisation that enables Africans to access health services, information, support and skills opportunities' (AISD 2013). AISD has been working in health promotion in Nottingham for over five years, especially within the area of HIV health promotion. African Health Celebration events have aimed to increase awareness of HIV and testing, late testing being a key issue within the African communities in the UK. The events also addressed the stigma, denial and fear associated with HIV. But rather than making the events solely about HIV, it was decided to raise awareness of health issues in general, especially those of concern to the African community. Amdani Juma, the director of AISD, feels that these events work because they give health professionals a chance to interact one-to-one with the African community on different health issues, and people are able to get mini health checks for diabetes, blood pressure and sexual health screening. He feels events such as these increase health literacy and the confidence of the community with regard to accessing health services. It is important that the events take place in community venues rather than clinical venues, making them more accessible. Amdani also believes that these events help to tackle social isolation. Individuals coming to a new country can feel very isolated, which can lead to depression, so these events bring people together to eat, talk and make connections and to start to come out physically and mentally, which is a positive for their mental health.

## Conclusion

This chapter has provided a background to BME communities in the UK, examined key health inequalities affecting those communities and considered whether there is a need for specific services for BME communities. Speaking to local professionals, there is a consensus that there is a need for services to be culturally competent. Staff need to be more aware of diversity. This does not mean that all people with a certain characteristic need to be treated a certain way, rather cultural awareness gives a background with which to work. This can be achieved by educating staff in the experiences of different communities, addressing stereotypes and providing practical knowledge; for example, regarding how to access and use interpreting services effectively. Promoting person-centred care ensures individuals are treated according to need. Most people would agree that all should be treated equally. Some specific BME services are needed, but for most health issues people should receive equal treatment at the point of contact. This is everyone's responsibility, from the reception desk to the consultant. This chapter also gave examples of successful health promotion activities aimed at BME communities to address health inequalities and to improve health for a group that has experienced these inequalities over decades. These examples are key because they have been delivered by knowledgeable, experienced and dedicated people in the community. Such practitioners continue to learn and have a duty to share that success with others.

I would like to thank all the contributors to this chapter:

Lisa Robinson – Bright Ideas Nottingham
Dr Chris Udenze – NDU (Life) Surgery
Kinsi Clarke – Into the Mainstream
Amdani Juma – African Institute for Social Development

## References

AISD (African Institute for Social Development) (2013) Website: http://www.africaninstitute.org.uk/.

BHF (British Heart Foundation) (2013a) *Cardiovascular Disease*. Available online: http://www.bhf.org.uk/heart-health/conditions/cardiovascular-disease.aspx.

BHF (British Heart Foundation) (2013b) *Your Ethnicity and Heart Disease*. Available online: http://www.bhf.org.uk/heart-health/prevention/ethnicity.aspx.

BME Cancer Communities (2013) Website: http://bmecancer.com/.

Cancer Equality UK. Website: http://www.cancerequality.co.uk/.

CHAI (Commission for Healthcare Audit and Inspection) (2005) *Count Me In: Results of a national census of inpatients in mental health hospitals and facilities in England and Wales*.

DH (Department of Health) (1992) *The Health of the Nation: A strategy for health in England*. London: HMSO.

DH (Department of Health) (2012) *Guidance on Providing NHS Treatment for Asylum Seekers and Refugees*. Available online: https://www.gov.uk/government/news/guidance-on-providing-nhs-treatment-for-asylum-seekers-and-refugees.

Diabetes UK (2010) *Key Statistics on Diabetes*. Available online: http://www.diabetes.org.uk/Documents/Reports/Diabetes_in_the_UK_2010.pdf

Fitzpatrick, M. (2005) 'Profiling mental health needs: What about your Irish patients?' *British Journal of General Practice* (October).

FPH (Faculty of Public Health) (2008) *The Health Needs of Asylum Seekers*. London: Faculty of Public Health. Available online: http://www.fph.org.uk/uploads/bs_aslym_seeker_health.pdf.

*The Guardian* (2012) 'Black and minority ethnic mental health patients "marginalised" under coalition'. 17 April 2012.

Harrison, G. (2002) 'Ethnic minorities and the Mental Health Act'. *The British Journal of Psychiatry* 180: 198–9.

He, J., Klag, M.J., Appel, L.J., Charleston, J. and Whelton, P.K. (1999) 'The renin-angiotensin system and blood pressure: Differences between blacks and whites'. *American Journal of Hypertension* 12(6): 555–62.

HPA (Health Protection Agency) (2005) *HIV Diagnoses by Ethnic Group: England, Wales and Northern Ireland*.

Lane, D.A. and Lip, G.Y.H. (2001) 'Ethnic differences in hypertension and blood pressure control in the UK'. *QJM: An International Journal of Medicine* 94(7): 391–6.

Marmot, M. (2010) *Fair Society, Healthy Lives: The Marmot Review: Strategic review of health inequalities in England post-2010*.

Mental Health Foundation (2013) *Black and Minority Ethnic Communities*. Available online: www.mentalhealth.org.uk/help-information/mental-health-a-z/B/BME-communities/.

The Migration Observatory (2013) *Long-Term International Migration Flows to and from the UK*. Available online: http://www.migrationobservatory.ox.ac.uk/sites/files/migobs/

Briefing%20-%20Long%20Term%20Migration%20Flows%20to%20and%20from%20
20the%20UK_0.pdf.

NAT (National AIDS Trust) (2013) *Black Africans*. Available online: http://www.nat.org.
uk/HIV-Facts/Statistics/Latest-UK-statistics/Black-Africans.aspx.

Netto, G., Bhopal, R., Lederle, N., Khatoon, J. and Jackson, A. (2010) 'How can health
promotion interventions be adapted for minority ethnic communities? Five principles for
guiding the development of behavioural interventions'. *Health Promotion International*
25(2): 248–57.

Newcastle Joint Strategic Needs Assessment (2013) Available online: http://www.
newcastlejsna.org.uk/book/export/html/1013.

The NHS Constitution (2012) Available online: http://www.nhs.uk/choiceinthenhs/
rightsandpledges/nhsconstitution/pages/overview.aspx.

The NHS Handbook to the Constitution (2013) Available online: http://www.nhs.uk/
choiceintheNHS/Rightsandpledges/NHSConstitution/Documents/2013/handbook-to-
the-nhs-constitution.pdf.

ONS (Office for National Statistics) (2011) *Life Expectancy at Birth and at Age 65 by
Local Areas in the United Kingdom, 2004–06 to 2008–10*. Newport: Office for National
Statistics.

PHE (Public Health England) (2013) *Ethnic Minority Health*. Available online: http://www.
apho.org.uk/resource/browse.aspx?RID=78571.

RCOG (Royal College of Obstetricians and Gynaecologists) (2004) *Confidential Enquiry
in Maternal and Child Health: Why mothers die 2000–2002*. The sixth report of the
confidential enquiry into maternal deaths in the UK. London: RCOG.

Thompson, R. (2013) *Here Me Now: The uncomfortable reality of prostate cancer in Afro-
Caribbean men*. BME Cancer Communities.

UK Government (2010) *The Equality Act UK*. Available online: http://www.legislation.
gov.uk/ukpga/2010/15/contents.

UK Government (2012) *Ethnicity and National Identity in England and Wales 2011*. Available online: http://www.ons.gov.uk/ons/rel/census/2011-census/key-statistics-for-local-
authorities-in-england-and-wales/rpt-ethnicity.html.

UNHCR (2013) *The Facts: Asylum in the UK*. Available online: http://www.unhcr.org.
uk/about-us/the-uk-and-asylum.html.

University of Leeds (2013) *More Ethnically Diverse Populations For UK Local Areas*.
Available online: http://www.leeds.ac.uk/news/article/3354/more_ethnically_diverse_
populations_for_uk_local_areas.

# 9 Focus on mental health promotion, obesity and alcohol

*Vicky Baldwin,
Anne Pridgeon and
Stephanie James*

## MENTAL HEALTH PROMOTION: PRINCIPLES FOR EFFECTIVE PRACTICE

### Introduction

There are many different perspectives regarding mental health promotion and the role it plays within health care and wider services. Forsman *et al.* (2011) argue that it can be seen in two ways, first as the promotion of positive mental health, and second as the prevention of ill health, whether at a primary, secondary or tertiary level. Rather than offering a theoretical debate as to what the concept is, this chapter will explore a practice-based approach to mental health promotion. The key aspects of mental health promotion, including core principles to support interventions, will be reviewed to provide a framework for developing strategies. Examples of interventions will also be provided to demonstrate mental health promotion in practice.

### Mental health promotion

Traditionally mental health promotion has been viewed as any action that aims to enhance the mental well-being of individuals, families, organisations and communities (DH 2001). Mental health promotion has been on the national agenda for a number of years, and in 2001 the Department of Health recognised the need for mental health promotion, making it standard in their new National Service Framework on Mental Health, thereby prioritising action on mental health promotion. Since then, a number of key policy documents have been released emphasising the importance of mental health promotion (DH 2001, 2003, 2011a; Department of Mental Health 2006). It is important to consider the preventative role that mental health promotion plays in supporting long-term mental health in those individuals not experiencing mental health difficulties as well as the wider community. Barry and Jenkins (2007) identify that mental health promotion is concerned with achieving positive mental health and supporting quality of life. This is relevant to all individuals, communities and societies and therefore interventions and approaches should be focused on more than an individual level. There is an opportunity for mental health promotion to work in an educational capacity to help develop understanding of mental health issues as well as supporting positive mental health overall. In light of this, mental health promotion should be seen as the responsibility of all health and social care professionals, not just those working within the mental health field.

It has been suggested that mental health promotion is the same as health promotion but with a focus on mental health rather than physical health (Cattan and Tilford 2006). However, there is now a growing consensus for the need to integrate mental health into the wider health promotion agenda. In a health care field that is moving towards an integrated model of delivery, interventions need to respond to this by focusing on a combination of physical and mental health issues. The cross-government paper, *No Health without Mental Health* (DH 2011a), also sent a clear message regarding the need to place an emphasis on the importance of mental health. Mental health promotion provides an opportunity to explore the issues most relevant to an individual, community or the wider society, whether they be mental health or physical health, or, in many cases, a combination of the two.

## Promotion and prevention

There are a range of perspectives on the role of promotion and prevention in the health promotion field. Cattan and Tilford (2006) highlight that in fact by promoting positive mental health there are preventative benefits in reducing mental health difficulties. Jané-Llopis *et al.* (2010) argue that mental health promotion encompasses both prevention and promotion and therefore interventions should be developed with this in mind. This indicates the need for a whole systems approach to considering mental health promotion. For example, when delivering interventions within a school setting, the focus should be on both promoting the mental health of young people, teachers and the wider school staff and exploring opportunities to prevent mental health difficulties either developing or continuing through increasing access to services when needed. This requires a more dynamic response to delivering interventions, ensuring that such interventions are informed by an understanding of the context and the individuals involved.

## What are mental health promotion interventions?

Mental health promotion interventions cover a diversity of issues and can be delivered in a variety of forms, whether it be educationally focused at an individual level or a national approach aimed at reducing the stigma associated with mental health. Table 9.1 provides examples of mental health promotion interventions focused at primary, secondary and national levels.

## Models of mental health promotion

There are a number of models of health promotion focused on identifying different factors to consider when designing or implementing interventions. Many of these have

Table 9.1 Mental health promotion interventions

| | | |
|---|---|---|
| Primary | • Increase understanding<br>• Prevent mental health difficulties<br>• Reduce stigma<br>• Improve individual motivation and self-esteem<br>• Reduce mental health symptoms | • Increased help-seeking behavior<br>• Development of self-management strategies<br>• Increase in self-esteem resulting in increased motivation | • Online resources for primary care staff aimed at developing understanding and awareness of particular mental health issues<br>• Coping skills workshops for individuals experiencing anxiety and depression in the community |
| Secondary | • Develop understanding and awareness<br>• Reduce mental health symptoms<br>• Increase personal responsibility for health<br>• Support appropriate access to services | • Increased awareness of protective and risk factors<br>• Enhanced ability to manage mental health symptoms<br>• Increased engagement with services | • Healthy eating classes within a medium secure mental health unit focused on managing obesity whilst improving psychological well-being<br>• Goals-based motivational interviewing to support treatment access and engagement |
| Regional or national | • Develop national awareness and understanding of mental health<br>• Reduce stigma associated with mental health<br>• Promote healthy behaviour<br>• Enhance acceptance within communities<br>• Increase access to support | • Increased understanding of mental health difficulties and how to access support<br>• Reduction in stigma<br>• Increased social engagement in mental health | • Mental health first aid training focused on increasing understanding of mental health and participants' ability to signpost individuals to services where appropriate. Further information can be accessed via http://www.mhfaengland.org/<br>• Time to Change national mental health campaign supporting a range of projects and interventions, see www.time-to-change.org.uk |

been used to explore mental health promotion and have relevance in the field. Examples include Downie *et al.*'s (1990) model of health promotion, which talks of three overlapping spheres of activity: health education, health protection and prevention. Although this model attempts to cover all aspects of health promotion there is little emphasis on the responsibility of the individual. As Prochaska and DiClemente (1984) highlight in their stages of change model, even if a health promotion activity would provide great benefits to individuals, the knowledge of this alone is often not enough to actually make changes. Whilst most individuals will go through the different stages of change, they argue that the key to interventions being successful is motivation of the individual. This factor of motivation tends to be missed in many models of health promotion. In light of this, interventions must consider the individual as well as the wider target group. One of the most helpful models focused specifically on mental health promotion is that offered by Barry and Jenkins (2007). The Generic Template for Action provides four key stages in implementing mental health promotion, with useful guidance on the practicalities of each stage. Health promotion and mental health promotion models themselves, although offering helpful suggestions and useful themes, do not always provide health promoters with a clear idea of how to design and implement a mental health promotion intervention. The model may offer direction in terms of areas to develop or concepts to consider in approaching a strategy; however, there can be limited practical advice and support relating to what to actually deliver. This is where the Barry and Jenkins (2007) model can be of use to provide a clearly defined structure for implementation in practice.

Given the diverse views and perspectives within the mental health field, the role of models can also vary depending on the context and the target group. Models can be used to inform thinking about an approach and help to develop ideas; however, a model alone is not enough to develop an intervention. The most helpful form of support in developing and delivering mental health promotion interventions is the use of underpinning core principles to inform and direct the work. Seedhouse (2003) supports this notion, indicating that most health promotion is produced from unrealistic goals and is too rigid in its structure to produce accurate results. He emphasises within his Rational Field's model the importance of identifying key values, classifications and instincts. By identifying these aspects we are able to explore our own thinking and our policies in a more open-minded manner. These values and principles can then be combined with the use of a model or template, if appropriate, to support the practitioner or worker to undertake the interventions effectively.

## Key principles of effective mental health promotion

As described above, establishing core principles to support mental health promotion can provide the greatest support in the development and implementation process. The following core principles, although not an exhaustive list, can be used to guide practice and ensure all aspects of an approach are considered:

- Understanding the service user/target group and choosing an appropriate method
- Sustainability
- Service user co-production

- Partnership working
- Utilising evidence and measuring outcomes.

## Understanding the service user/target group

Understanding the target group for mental health promotion interventions is perhaps the first and most important principle. Identifying the target population and then exploring how to engage effectively takes careful consideration. For some interventions, targeting a particular high-risk group may be relevant, or alternatively the focus may be on a whole population. Determining this will make a difference to the method and approach taken for the intervention. Mental health promotion has a role to play across the life span and therefore consideration should be given to all age groups (Royal College of Psychiatrists 2010). There has been increasing focus over recent years on targeting young people and parenting with evidence of successful outcomes (Essler *et al.* 2006). This is supported by the evidence indicating that first onset of mental health experiences occurs in childhood (Kessler *et al.* 2007). There is also growing evidence for the need to focus on older adults within an ageing population. Forsman *et al.* (2011), in their study of the use of psychosocial interventions in the promotion of mental health in older adults, found positive results, including a reduction in symptoms and an increase in positive mental health experiences. Therefore, interventions can be focused at any age depending on the overall aims and intended outcomes; however, in deciding on a target group, consideration should be given to:

- The evidence available regarding previous interventions and their effectiveness with particular age groups
- The method and approach used and the appropriateness of this for different age groups (e.g. are online activities the most appropriate choice for individuals who may not have access to the internet?)
- Accessibility needs of individuals/communities involved
- Social and demographic factors
- Local context for delivery.

The above factors should be considered when identifying an approach, but careful attention should be given to the impact of targeting specific groups and the potential for stigmatisation, for example in targeting low income or deprived populations. It is also important to consider when targeting specific diagnoses or difficulties that other appropriate groups and individuals are not excluded from beneficial interventions.

## Sustainability

Sustainability is another key factor to consider when developing mental health promotion programmes. The challenge of delivering interventions can often be related to resource and time implications and therefore sustainability should be embedded into any programme strategy. For example, in the Let's Talk About It project described in the case study later, sustainability was generated through educating teachers to deliver follow-up interventions. This negated the school from having to keep paying for performances, yet enabled it to make use of the learning long-term. Other ways to support sustainability include identifying opportunities for generating self-funding streams. Knapp *et al.* (2011), in their review of interventions, found that mental health promotion interventions have the ability to become self-financing over time, which supports the long-term outcomes of the work. There are also other benefits of developing sustainability, including increasing motivation and engagement within target groups. Where possible, if individuals or communities can take on responsibility for the work, this may result in a sense of ownership, which in itself may have positive mental health benefits. Individuals may also feel empowered to address wider issues or work more collaboratively to support the sustainability of a project.

## Service user co-production

There is a wealth of evidence in the mental health field supporting the need for effective service user involvement (Tait and Lester 2005; British Psychological Society 2008; Bracken and Thomas 2009; Tritter 2009; Martin and Finn 2011). More recently, there has been a move to working with service users within a co-production model rather than purely involvement. This model advocates for the equal involvement and engagement of service users in the planning, development and delivery of interventions. Co-production places an emphasis on a collaborative model of working rather than 'involving' service users at points within a project. Bovaird (2007) argues that there is a need to move away from traditional thinking around the role of service users and rethink our approach to working in a co-production capacity. In the field of mental health promotion service users have a key role to play at all stages. Service users and practitioners must work together in the development of interventions, allowing service users to inform the approach with their experiences and offer expertise regarding what works with particular groups. Needham (2008) reinforces the need for collective dialogue and deliberation between co-producers to support the work. Key issues to take into account when co-producing with service users include:

- Effective recruitment to ensure representative experience is linked to the focus of the intervention
- Clarity about roles and responsibilities
- Ensuring appropriate payment for the role
- Support and training
- Feedback.

These aspects will support an effective model of working together whilst ensuring clarity regarding the practicalities and boundaries is managed.

## Partnership working

There are many benefits to partnership working in the delivery of mental health promotion interventions. Seeking to establish a range of experiences and approaches will enhance the overall method adopted. Partnerships involve identifying the most relevant stakeholders and establishing what involvement they may be able to have in the approach. Barry and Jenkins (2007) highlight the importance of establishing partnerships to enhance the support for the mental health promotion intervention. Partnerships may include local community groups, individual stakeholders or organisations with key skills or strengths to support the project. Partnerships may also be created with local and national service user organisations to strengthen the opportunities for co-production. In order to support effective partnership working, plans and agreements must be put in place to create clarity about the different partner roles and responsibilities. It may also be helpful to establish a forum or steering group with appropriate representation across the partners to help drive the interventions. In small-scale mental health promotion interventions, partners may be limited to different disciplines or staff groups within an organisation. Whether the partnership is small or large, establishing a model for working is crucial to support the long-term development of the project.

## Evidence and outcomes

Establishing the evidence base for an intervention is an important stage of mental health promotion. Exploring where activities have already been successful and the outcomes of this is crucial. A number of reviews of the effectiveness of interventions have been undertaken which demonstrate a wide variety of outcomes and learning (Forsman *et al.* 2011; Taylor *et al.* 2007; Tennant *et al.* 2007; Jané-Llopis *et al.* 2005). These reviews, along with others, provide useful information regarding key learning in the implementation and changes for future delivery, which may be useful in informing an approach. When discussing the evidence for mental health promotion, it is also important in this financial climate to consider the economic view. Considerable work is being undertaken to explore the financial impact of mental health promotion and as a result the economic case is growing substantially (Knapp *et al.* 2011; Zechmeister *et al.* 2008; Friedli and Parsonage 2007). Research into the economic impact indicates both value for money and the ability of interventions to generate a wide range of outcomes at an individual and community level (Knapp *et al.* 2011). Evaluation strategies and methods should therefore focus on capturing a broad range of outcomes, including the economic impact where possible. Evaluation approaches should be contextualised to the activity and the target group with a range of methods being used to access the most accurate data. Where possible, previously validated tools can be used, or alternatively work should be undertaken to establish the most appropriate format to generate and measure outcomes. As with the intervention, the focus should be on a whole systems approach, taking into account all stakeholders related to the project.

## Summary

As this section has demonstrated, mental health promotion can take many forms and target a range of groups. The importance of engaging with the interventions using core principles has been explored to support the delivery of context-specific, evidence-based strategies. With an increasing national focus on mental health, it is clear that mental health promotion is the responsibility of all, whether it be focused on a one-to-one individual level or working nationally. Practitioners should consider their responsibility in promoting mental health alongside current practice and ensure both promotion and prevention is taken into account.

## Mental health promotion community case study: The Let's Talk About It project

The Let's Talk About It project is delivered in partnership between Nottinghamshire Healthcare NHS Trust, the Institute of Mental Health Nottingham, local theatre and creative consultants. The project is an innovative model for delivering a whole systems approach to mental health promotion within the school setting. The project aims to support the emotional health and well-being of young people in schools through delivering interventions to young people and school staff. The project has a key focus on raising awareness about mental health and challenging stigma amongst young people. The key components of the project include:

- A 60-minute interactive theatre performance based on the story of two young people both experiencing mental health difficulties. Interactive approaches are used during the performance to engage the young people and to highlight key issues that may impact on mental health and coping strategies that can support mental health, including accessing support services.
- Prior to the theatre performance, a developmental session is delivered with staff working in the schools aimed at developing an understanding of mental health, exploring the focus of the performance and equipping the staff to deliver long-term follow-up interventions. Staff are provided with a follow-up lesson plan with experiential activities relating to the theatre performance to be used as a follow-up session and as an ongoing resource.
- Alongside the performance, young people are also given pocket-sized information handouts signposting students to the best places to look for help and support if they are experiencing difficulties with their mental health.

The project has been delivered in over twelve schools within Nottinghamshire and has reached over 2,000 young people and 80 staff. Baseline and follow-up data is collected from the young people, and the project has demonstrated positive outcomes, including an overall improvement in knowledge and understanding and an increase in help-seeking behaviour accessed through teachers as a first point of contact. Not only does the project help to support schools in promoting and subsequently preventing mental health difficulties, it also seeks to help schools respond to many aspects of national school requirements and evidence-based best practice

## OBESITY

This specific section considers the issue of excess weight and discusses the evidence base along with practical examples of interventions that are currently being used.

## Obesity as a public health issue

Excess weight (being overweight or obese) is essentially caused by eating and drinking more calories than are used up each day over a long period of time, leading to an accumulation of body fat. It is a leading cause of type 2 diabetes, heart disease and cancer, and not only does it affect physical health, it contributes to poor mental health and reduced quality of life (Butland *et al*. 2007). Ultimately it places a national financial burden in terms of health and social care costs on employers through lost productivity, and on families because of the increasing numbers of those experiencing long-term conditions that lead to disability and early death. Children who are overweight or obese are more likely to become obese adults and are developing at a much earlier age those obesity-related conditions normally seen in adulthood, such as type 2 diabetes (Board of Science 2005). Obesity during pregnancy (maternal obesity) is also increasingly being seen as a public health issue, as this increases childhood obesity and infant mortality as well as impacting on the mother's immediate and future health (CMACE 2010). Certain population groups are more at risk of excess weight and there are key stages in life when people are more likely to put on weight (Butland *et al*. 2007). Groups at risk include those from lower socio-economic and socially disadvantaged groups, particularly women, Caucasian and Bangladeshi populations, and those with physical disabilities, learning disabilities or severe and enduring mental illness such as schizophrenia or bipolar disease (Butland *et al*. 2007). The key stages when people are likely to put on weight are:

- Men in their late 30s
- Women entering long-term relationships
- Women during and after pregnancy
- Women at menopause
- People who give up smoking
- People who retire
- People suffering from psychological problems such as stress, depression and anxiety.

(SIGN 2010)

Sustained modest weight loss of 5–10 kg or 5–10 per cent reduction of body weight at one year is associated with:

- Improved lipid profiles
- Reduced osteoarthritis-related disability
- Lowered all-cause, cancer and diabetes mortality in some patient groups
- Reduced blood pressure
- Improved glycaemic control
- Reduction in risk of developing type 2 diabetes
- Improved lung function in patients in asthma (SIGN 2010).

SIGN (2010) states that weight loss targets should be based on the individual's co-morbidities and risks rather than just weight alone, and that for those with a BMI greater than 35 and associated obesity-related comorbidities a weight loss of greater than

15–20 per cent will be needed to obtain a sustained improvement in comorbidities. The guidance concludes that the aim of weight loss and weight maintenance interventions should be to:

- Improve pre-existing obesity-related comorbidities
- Reduce the future risk of obesity related comorbidities
- Improve physical, mental and social well-being.

The national strategy 'Healthy Lives, Healthy People: A call to action on obesity in England' (DH 2011b) takes a life course approach to tackling and managing excess weight by transforming the environment so that it encourages healthy lifestyles while providing support on diet and physical activity for those that need to lose weight. This strategy has two national ambitions:

1. A sustained downward trend in the level of excess weight in children by 2020.
2. A downward trend in the level of excess weight averaged across all adults by 2020.

From April 2013, top tier local government through the transfer of public health became responsible for the implementation of the National Child Measurement Programme (NCMP) and the provision of local obesity interventions (excluding bariatric surgery), including nutrition and physical activity initiatives. The new Public Health Outcomes Framework (PHOF) has a number of indicators (Box 9.1) relating to adult and childhood obesity that will be used to measure progress in tackling excess weight at a local level (DH 2012a).

Established in 2005, the National Child Measurement Programme (NCMP) is an annual programme that measures the height and weight of children upon starting

---

### *Box 9.1* Public health outcome indicators relating to adult and childhood obesity

**Domain 1: Improving the wider determinants of health**

- Utilisation of green space for exercise/health reasons

**Domain 2: Health improvement**

- Breastfeeding
- Excess weight in 4–5- and 10–11-year-olds (from the National Child Measurement Programme data)
- Excess weight in adults (national data from Health Survey of England and local authority data to be collected using the Active People's Survey)
- Diet
- Proportion of physically active and inactive adults

school (aged 4–5) and in Year 6 (aged 10–11). Its purpose is to provide local population level surveillance data on the weight status of children to allow analysis of trends in weight that will then inform the planning and delivery of services for children. Parents or carers are given information regarding their child's weight and signposted to services for support and advice (DH 2012b).

Local data on excess weight in adults is not routinely collected and therefore estimates using national data from the Health Survey of England have traditionally been used; however, in the future local authority data will be collected using the Active People's Survey (DH 2012b).

## The evidence base for weight loss

The current evidence base of what works in the prevention and treatment of excess weight is limited. The National Obesity Observatory has summarised the evidence from NICE and the Cochrane Collaboration for the prevention of childhood obesity (National Obesity Observatory 2009) and treatment of adult (Cavill and Ells 2010) and child obesity (Ells and Cavill 2009). There is limited evidence of effective approaches to preventing child obesity; however, it recommends that 'programmes should be multi-component interventions, ideally addressing diet and physical activity together and should involve family and peer support where possible using behavioural programmes aimed at changing diet and physical activity' (Ells and Cavill 2009).

For the treatment of obesity in adults and children a range of lifestyle interventions are considered effective:

- Multi-component, tailored interventions that focus on diet and physical activity together rather than attempting to modify either diet or physical activity alone.
- Physical activity interventions that focus on activities which fit easily into people's everyday lives and are tailored to people's individual preferences and circumstances.
- Dietary interventions that aim to improve diet and reduce energy intake and involve dietary modification, targeted advice and family involvement and goal setting.
- Behavioural interventions for adults that include self-monitoring, stimulus control and goal setting.

Current NICE guidance documents related to obesity, diet and physical activity are given in Box 9.2.

This guidance suggests the need to tackle elements of the environment that do not promote a healthy lifestyle and are 'obesity-promoting' whilst encouraging improvements in diet and physical activity levels at an individual level. NICE is currently developing guidance on managing overweight and obesity in children and young people through lifestyle weight management services and managing overweight and obesity in adults through lifestyle weight management services. Frontline health and social care staff need to have the skills and knowledge to raise the issue of excess weight and signpost to local services, therefore 'making every contact count' (NHS Futures Forum 2012). Brief interventions are limited by time and focused on changing behaviour and can lead to short-term changes in behaviour and body weight if they:

---

### *Box 9.2* **Current NICE guidance documents related to obesity, diet and physical activity**

Obesity: the prevention, identification, assessment and management of over-weight and obesity in adults and children (2006) CG43

Four commonly used methods to increase physical activity: Brief interventions in primary care, exercise referral schemes, pedometers and community based exercise programmes for walking and cycling (2006) PH02

Behaviour change (2007) PH07

Physical activity and the environment (2008) PH08

Maternal and child nutrition (2008) PH11

Promoting physical activity in the workplace (2008) PH13

Promoting physical activity in children and young people (2009) PH17

Prevention of cardiovascular disease (2010) PH25

Weight management before, during and after pregnancy (2010) PH27

Preventing type 2 diabetes – population and community interventions (2011) PH35

Walking and cycling (2012) PH41

Obesity: Working with local communities (2012) PH42

Physical activity: Brief advice for adults in primary care (2013)

---

- Focus on both diet and physical activity
- Are delivered by practitioners trained in motivational interviewing
- Incorporate behavioural techniques such as self-monitoring
- Are tailored to individual circumstances
- Encourage the individual or patient to seek support from other people.

(National Obesity Forum 2011)

## Surgical methods of weight loss

Bariatric surgery is the name for weight loss surgery which is recommended by NICE as a treatment option for people with morbid obesity. This is classified as those individuals who have a high body mass index (BMI) along with other significant disease such as type 2 diabetes or high blood pressure that could be improved if they lost weight. Surgery is only considered appropriate for adults with morbid obesity when all relevant non-surgical approaches have been unsuccessful. It is not recommended for children and adolescents (NICE 2006). The cost-effectiveness appears to be greatest in those with a BMI greater than 40 and for those with a BMI greater than 30 with type 2 diabetes (Picot *et al.* 2009).

## Maintaining weight loss

Research suggests that approximately 20 per cent of overweight individuals can lose approximately 10 per cent of their body weight intentionally and maintain this at one year (Wing and Phelan 2005). The National Weight Control Registry (2013), established in 1994 in the USA, is the largest prospective organisation investigating long-term successful weight loss maintenance. An average of 33 kg has been lost by members with sustained weight losses for more than five years (Klem *et al.* 1997). Six key strategies have been identified that may support long-term weight loss maintenance:

- High levels of physical activity – one hour of moderate-intensity activity daily
- A diet low in calories and fat
- Having breakfast
- Regular self-monitoring of weight
- A consistent eating pattern
- Preventing slips from turning into larger regains.

(Klem *et al.* 1997)

## Current interventions used to tackle excess weight

Given the above evidence base, many areas have adopted a four-tiered prevention and management of excess weight model.

### Tier 1: Primary prevention and early interventions

The prevention of weight gain starting in childhood offers the most effective means of achieving healthy weight in the population. A partnership approach is needed that recognises that weight can be influenced by a broad variety of environmental and community factors. Activity at this level should create environments that actively promote healthy lifestyles and address the 'obesity promoting' environment and will make the greatest contribution to longer-term changes in the numbers of individuals with excess weight. Interventions that aim to prevent and provide early intervention to tackle excess weight at a national or local population include:

- Active transport policies and initiatives to reduce car dependency and promote cycling and walking
- Spatial planning policies to limit the numbers of hot fast food outlets in an area
- Schools, workplaces and community settings promoting healthy eating and an increase in physical activity
- Promotion of leisure and green space and exercise referral schemes that target those who are sedentary
- Promotion of breast feeding and the UNICEF Baby Friendly Initiative (BFI) accreditation (UNICEF 2013)
- Food and nutrition initiatives such as food education and skills (cook and eat), healthy eating catering awards and calorie information on restaurant menus
- Social marketing campaigns such as Change for Life (Kirkby 2013; NHS 2013a).

## Tier 2: Community-based weight management services

This tier is the provision of a community-based lifestyle/weight management service for those who are already overweight or obese. Targeting these services can help to address the inequalities in excess weight rates between population groups and ensure the best use of resources. These services tend to offer a programme lasting 12 weeks along with reviews at 6- and 12-month periods. Many different areas across the country now commission community-based lifestyle/weight management services for both adults and children.

## Tier 3: Specialist multidisciplinary weight management service

This tier is aimed at the provision of a specialist multidisciplinary weight management service for those individuals with longstanding and complex obesity. The composition of teams varies from area to area, but may include doctors, psychologists, dieticians and exercise practitioners. At this tier the use of anti-obesity drugs may be considered in adults aged over 18 years after dietary, exercise and behavioural approaches have been started and evaluated.

## Tier 4: Weight loss (bariatric) surgery

This tier is the provision of specialised complex obesity services and includes weight loss (bariatric) surgery for those with morbid obesity. Following the Health and Social Care Act 2012 (DH 2012c), NHS England is responsible for the commissioning of bariatric surgery.

# Conclusion

This section has provided an overview of the current available evidence base and associated interventions to tackle excess weight. It must be acknowledged that the evidence base of what works to prevent and manage excess weight is currently limited. There is a need for both commissioners and providers of services to ensure that high quality, consistent evaluation of weight management, physical activity and dietary interventions that measures a range of outcomes and impacts is undertaken in order to improve the evidence base for the future.

# ALCOHOL CONSUMPTION

## Alcohol as a public health issue

Alcohol-related hospital admissions in England doubled in the ten years from 2002/03 (510,700 admissions) to 2011/12 (1,220,300 admissions) despite a national downturn in alcohol intake. Excess alcohol consumption is thought to cost the NHS £3.5 billion every year (NHS 2013b). Alcohol use is ranked according to the impact it can have on an individual's health; 'low risk' (less than 2–3 units per day for a woman, 3–4 units a day for a man), 'increasing risk' (more than 2–3 units a day for a woman, more than 3–4 units a day for a man), 'high risk' (more than 35 units per week for a woman, more than 50 units a week for a man) and 'dependency'. 'Binge drinking' (drinking twice the daily guidance in one session) stretches across all categories. The Department of Health currently advises that women drink no more than 2–3 units a day on a regular basis and men no more than 3–4 units a day on a regular basis (this guidance is for adults, there is separate guidance for under-18s) with at least 48 hours abstinence following a heavy drinking session. The majority of people in the UK drink responsibly, and in 2006 The General Household Survey estimated that 24.8 million people drink at 'low risk', 7.6 million at 'increasing risk' and 2.9 million at 'high risk'. Men drinking at 'increasing risk' levels are four times as likely to develop high blood pressure, women twice as likely to be hypertensive and both sexes are 13 times more likely to develop liver disease (Anderson 2007).

Alcohol misuse is no respecter of social position and can affect anyone from the stereotypical street drinker to academic professors. The impact of alcohol is also far-reaching, affecting families, friends, employment and the wider community. Alcohol is a legal 'drug' and due to the current UK licencing laws is available in a large number of places for a lengthy number of hours. The public can become confused due to this seemingly mixed message of ready availability and low price conflicting with harm to health. Moderate and controlled alcohol consumption is not harmful to health (Ronksley *et al.* 2011). Unlike with smoking cessation where people are told that they must stop completely, the health education message regarding alcohol consumption is not complete abstinence, instead people are advised to reduce their alcohol intake to acceptable levels. The exception to this message is for those individuals where it is considered that abstinence is the only way to address alcohol misuse. Abstinence from alcohol is the only option for some people, many of whom have tried controlled drinking without success or have medical conditions that require abstinence. Delivering a complex message can cause some confusion with the general public and result in all messages being ignored; however, the majority of people need to simply reduce the amount they drink. In order to get the public to reduce their alcohol intake, health promotion campaigns throughout the 1980s and 1990s endeavoured to make the public aware of the amount of units contained in common alcoholic drinks, such as pints of beer, single measures of spirits, and so on. The benefit of this method was its relative simplicity. However, due to the vast range of alcoholic beverages now available and their different unit to volume ratios this message is now largely out of date. The general public generally aren't aware that the strength of alcoholic drinks on sale has increased significantly since the unit campaigns were initiated.

## Case study of alcohol awareness outreach service

### *The Last Orders alcohol prevention service*

The Last Orders alcohol service, funded by NHS Nottingham City and run by the charity Framework, has been part of Nottingham's alcohol landscape since 2009. It started as a primary care brief advice service and now provides the front door for alcohol services in Nottinghamshire with health promotion, training, specialist treatment and support services also part of the Last Orders brand.

From the outset Last Orders tried to be an accessible and inclusive service, aiming to be different from other alcohol services by not only focusing on dependent drinkers. A targeted approach was implemented with the aim of reaching increasing and high-risk drinkers along with groups that may not normally access an alcohol service. This made the link with alcohol health promotion much easier as the service was providing messages about cutting down rather than abstinence, although the service does signpost to abstinence-based services when appropriate.

Nottingham has higher-than-average alcohol-attributable hospital admissions with a high alcohol crime rate (Public Health England 2013); 57 per cent of citizens fall into the increasing/high risk categories of drinking compared with 30 per cent nationally (Nottingham City Council 2012). Nottingham is one of the most deprived areas in the country, ranked 20th out of 326 England districts (Nottingham City Council 2011) with high rates of health inequalities. It is understood that alcohol compounds existing health inequalities, so although a person living in a relatively wealthy part of the city may drink the same amount of alcohol as the person living in a more deprived part of the city, the person in the deprived area will die younger due to the cumulative health issues associated with health inequalities, such as poor diet and increased levels of smoking.

A combination of interventions is required in order to reduce the harm caused by alcohol, and Nottingham has made addressing alcohol harm one of its priorities with a strategy group addressing treatment, crime and harm prevention. People are most likely to change their behaviour if early intervention is used (NICE 2010). Screening tools are used across primary care to identify people at risk of alcohol harm and brief advice is given along with referrals to specialist alcohol services.

## The outreach service

Outreach services seek to engage with those hard-to-reach groups who are not in regular contact with mainstream services such as family doctors. Part of the outreach service is raising awareness of alcohol issues within the community by attendance and running stalls at health and community events throughout the city. The majority of people who come over to the stall are either in the pre-contemplation or contemplation stage of the Transtheoretical Model (Prochaska and DiClemente 1983). Those in the contemplation stage are aware they need to make some change to their drinking, but are often unsure what or how to change.

The first event Last Orders attended was the Lesbian, Gay, Bisexual and Transgender Pride event in July 2009. The initial intention was to promote the service to the local area, so leaflets were produced detailing the services provided. There was scepticism as to whether people would approach a stall dealing with alcohol consumption; however, it was decided to proceed and evaluate the interest. The day was a huge success, the weather was good and the stall ran out of materials after several hours. After this success it was decided to post a presence at further events and this increased the service's profile. Initially the stalls distributed 'Advice About Alcohol' leaflets, 'Drinking and You' booklets and alcohol calculators (drinks wheels). The leaflets and booklets were based on NHS materials, but contained local contacts and had Last Orders branding. The Last Orders branding was an important component in establishing the service across the city as it helped to give the new service identity. The colours used were also bright and had high impact to help the leaflets stand out. Last Orders decided to target family events and distribute 'freebies' in order to attract people to the stall such as pens, post-its and Last Orders-branded sweets in bags that also contained Last Orders information cards. Fake drinks designed to show units are displayed and are a hit in attracting people over to the stall, if only for them to ask if they are real. Once people come over to the stall staff engage them in discussions about alcohol units and have a brief chat about their drinking. The most recent additions to the stalls have been plastic unit measures and alcohol calorie wheels, as many people are interested in weight in relation to their health, but are not aware of the high calorific nature of alcohol. The Last Orders unit measures have proved to be very popular amongst the Nottingham City residents, with 200 given away at one event alone. The most important part of outreach is being non-judgemental and looking interested. This means trying to catch people's eye as they walk past and offering pens or just saying 'Hi'. It is important to allow people to browse and not to pressurise or 'hard sell' as there is so much stigma attached to alcohol. After a short while, a prop such as the drinks wheel can be used to engage the person in a conversation. The drinks wheel is a tool used to calculate an individual's unit intake; it may be good for staff to give themselves as an illustration, for example, 'When I go home tonight I will have one large glass of wine and that is three units'. Disclosing that staff also drink can again have the result of reducing stigma, relaxing the atmosphere and equalising the power dynamic. This encourages people to describe what they drink without the fear that they will 'be told off'. It opens the door for a longer discussion and brief advice. Most people aren't aware of the units they are drinking and also that some of the effects they are experiencing can be related back to their alcohol use. After giving brief advice the person can take some materials and can also take a longer workbook to work through. Research shows that 1 in 8 people approached will reduce their drinking (Kaner *et al.* 2007) and the SIPS trial (Kaner *et al.* 2013) showed that opportunistic brief advice has some of the best outcomes. Increasing awareness in the community means that the service gets known and gains a reputation for approachability. Currently Last Orders has a presence at events for parents, gypsy travellers, the Polish community, people with learning disabilities, people with hearing difficulties, people from the BME communities, students at colleges and universities and other community events, and has seen nearly 3,000 people to date.

The outreach part of Last Orders is, in relative terms, only a small part of what the service does, but has fast become the face of the service and as it is an integral part of the city's harm prevention plan, it should continue in the future.

## References

Anderson, P. (2007) *The Scale of Alcohol Related Harm*. London: Department of Health.
Barry, M. and Jenkins, R. (2007) *Implementing Mental Health Promotion*. London: Elsevier Limited.
Board of Science (2005) *Preventing Childhood Obesity*. London: British Medical Association.

Bovaird, T. (2007) 'Beyond engagement and participation: User and community coproduction of public services'. *Public Administration Review* 67(5): 846–60.

Bracken, P. and Thomas, P. (2009) 'Beyond consultation: The challenge of working with user/survivor and carer groups'. *The Psychiatrist* 33: 243–6.

British Psychological Society (2008) *Good Practice Guidelines: Service user and carer involvement within clinical psychology training*. Leicester: The British Psychological Society.

Butland, B., Jebb, S., Kopelman, P., McPherson, K., Thomas, S., Mardell, J. and Parry, V. (2007) *Foresight. Tackling Obesities: Future choices – project report*. London: Government Office for Science.

Cattan, M. and Tilford, S. (2006) *Mental Health Promotion*. Berkshire: Open University Press.

Cavill, N. and Ells, L. (2010) *Treating Adult Obesity through Lifestyle Change Interventions: A briefing paper for commissioners*. London: National Obesity Observatory.

CMACE (Centre for Maternal and Child Enquiries) (2010) *Maternal Obesity in the UK: Findings from a national project*. London: CMACE.

DH (Department of Health) (2001) *Making It Happen: A guide to delivering mental health promotion*. London: HMSO.

DH (Department of Health) (2003) 'Read the Signs': Mind Out for Mental Health Campaign. London: Department of Health.

DH (Department of Health) (2011a) *No Health without Mental Health: A cross-government mental health outcomes strategy*. London: Department of Health.

DH (Department of Health) (2011b) *Healthy Lives, Healthy People: A call to action on obesity in England*. London: Department of Health.

DH (Department of Health)/HIPD/PHDU (2012a) *Healthy Lives, Healthy People: Improving outcomes and supporting transparency*. London: Department of Health.

DH (Department of Health) (2012b) *National Child Measurement Programme Operational Guidance for the 2012/13 School Year*. London: Department of Health.

DH (Department of Health) (2012c) *Health and Social Care Act 2012*. London: Department of Health.

Department of Mental Health (2006) *Mental Health Futures Policy Paper: A vision for 2015*. London: HMSO.

Downie, R.S., Fyfe, C. and Tannahill, A. (1990) *Health Promotion: Models and values*. Oxford: Oxford University Press.

Ells, L. and Cavill, N. (2009) *Treating Childhood Obesity Through Lifestyle Change Interventions: A briefing paper for commissioners*. London: National Obesity Observatory.

Essler, V., Arthur, A. and Stickley, T. (2006) 'Using a school based intervention to challenge stigmatising attitudes'. *Journal of Mental Health* 15(2): 243–50.

Forsman, A.K., Nordmyr, J. and Wahlbeck, K. (2011) 'Psychosocial interventions for the promotion of mental health and the prevention of depression among older adults'. *Health Promotion International* 26(1): 85–107.

Friedli, L. and Parsonage, M. (2007) *Mental Health Promotion: Building an economic case*. Belfast: Northern Ireland Association for Mental Health.

Jané-Llopis, E., Barry, M., Hosman, C. and Patel, V. (2005) 'Mental health promotion works: A review'. *Promotion & Education* 12(9): 9–25.

Jané-Llopis, E., Katschnig, H., McDaid, D. and Wahlbeck, K. (2010) *Evidence in Public Mental Health – Commissioning, Interpreting and Making Use of Evidence on Mental Health Promotion and Mental Disorder Prevention: An everyday primer*. Lisbon: Instituto Nacional de Saúde Doutor Ricardo Jorge.

Kaner, E., Beter, F., Dickinson, H., Pienaar, E., Campbell, F., Schlesinger, C., *et al.* (2007) *Effectiveness of Brief Alcohol Interventions in Primary Care Populations.* Newcastle Upon Tyne: University of Newcastle.

Kaner, E., Bland, M., Cassidy, P., Coulton, S., Dale, V., Deluca, P., *et al.* (2013) 'Effectiveness of screening and brief alcohol intervention in primary care (SIPS trial): Pragmatic cluster randomised controlled trial'. *British Medical Journal* 346: e8501. doi: 10.1136/bmj.e8501.

Kessler, R.C., Amminger, G.P., Aguilar-Gaxiola, S., Alonso, J., Lee, S. and Üstün, T.B. (2007) 'Age of onset of mental disorders: A review of recent literature'. *Current Opinion Psychiatry* 20(4): 359–64.

Kirkby, T. (2013) 'Tackling obesity in cities'. *The Lancet Online.* 30 January 2013. Available online: http://download.thelancet.com/flatcontentassets/landia/pdfs/TLDE_NEWS_Kirby.pd.

Klem, M., Wing, R., McGuire, M., Seagle, H. and Hill, O. (1997) 'A descriptive study of individuals successful at long term maintenance of substantial weight loss'. *Amercian Journal of Clinical Nutrition* 66: 239–46.

Knapp, M., McDaid, D. and Parsonage, M. (2011) *Mental Health Promotion and Mental Illness Prevention: The economic case.* London: Department of Health.

Martin, G. and Finn, R. (2011) 'Patients as team members: Opportunities, challenges and paradoxes of including patients in multi-professional health-care teams'. *Sociology of Health & Illness* 33(7): 1050–65.

National Obesity Observatory (2009) *Preventing Childhood Obesity through Lifestyle Change Interventions.* London: National Obesity Observatory.

National Obesity Observatory (2011) *Brief Interventions for Weight Management.* London: National Obesity Observatory.

The National Weight Control Registry (2013) Available online: http://www.nwcr.ws/.

Needham, C. (2008) 'Realising the potential of co-production: Negotiating improvements in public services'. *Social Policy and Society* 7(2): 221–31.

NHS (2013a) *Change for Life.* Available online: http://www.nhs.uk/change4life/Pages/change-for-life.aspx.

NHS (2013b) *Statistics on Alcohol – England.* Leeds: The Health and Social Care Information Centre.

NHS Future Forum (2010) *The NHS's Role in the Public's Health.* London: Department of Health.

NICE (2006) *Obesity: The prevention, identification, assessment and management of overweight and obesity in adults and children* CG43. London: NICE.

NICE (2010) *Alcohol Use Disorders: Preventing harmful drinking.* London: NICE.

Nottingham City Council (2011) *The Indices Of Deprivation 2010: Compendium of results for Nottingham City.* Nottingham: Nottingham City Council.

Nottingham City Council (2012) *Joint Strategic Needs Assessment.* Nottingham: Nottingham City Council.

Picot, J., Jones, J., Colquitt, J.L., Gospodarevskaya, E., Loveman, E., Baxter, L. and Clegg, A.J. (2009) 'The clinical effectiveness and cost effectiveness of bariatric (weight loss) surgery for obesity: A systematic review and economic evaluation'. *Health Technology Assessment* 13(41).

Prochaska, J. and DiClemente, C. (1983) 'Stages and processes of self change of smoking: Towards an integrated model of change'. *Journal of Consultant Clinical Psychology* 51: 390–5.

Prochaska, J.O. and DiClemente, C.C. (1984) *The Transtheoretical Approach: Towards a systematic eclectic framework.* Homewood, IL: Dow Jones-Irwin.

Public Health England (2013) *Local Alcohol Profiles for England – Nottingham City*. London: Public Health England.

Ronksley, P., Brien, S., Turner, B., Mukamal, K. and Ghali, W. (2011) 'Association of alcohol consumption with selected cardiovascular disease outcomes: A systematic review and meta-analysis'. *British Medical Journal* 342: d671.

Royal College of Psychiatrists (2010) *No Health without Mental Health: The case for action*. Royal College of Psychiatrists Position statement PS4/2010. London: Royal College of Psychiatrists.

Seedhouse, D. (2003) *Total Health Promotion*. Chichester: John Wiley & Sons.

SIGN (Scottish Intercollegiate Guidelines Network) (2010) *Management of Obesity: A national clinical guideline*. Edinburgh: SIGN.

Tait, L. and Lester, H. (2005) 'Encouraging user involvement in mental health services'. *Advances in Psychiatric Treatment* 11: 168–75.

Taylor, L., Taske, N., Swann, C. and Waller, S. (2007) *Public Health Interventions to Promote Positive Mental Health and Prevent Mental Health Disorders Among Adults*. London: NICE.

Tennant, R., Goens, C., Barlow, J., Day, C. and Stewart-Brown, S. (2007) 'A systematic review of reviews of interventions to promote mental health and prevent mental health problems in children and young people'. *Journal of Public Mental Health* 6(1): 25–32.

Tritter, J. (2009) 'Revolution or evolution: The challenges of conceptualizing patient and public involvement in a consumerist world'. *Health Expectations* 12: 275–87.

UNICEF (2013) *Baby Friendly Initiative (BFI) accreditation*. Available online: http://www.unicef.org.uk/babyfriendly/.

Wing, R. and Phelan, S. (2005) 'Long term weight loss maintenance'. *Amercian Journal of Clinical Nutrition* 82: 222–5.

Zechmeister, I., Reinhold, K., McDaid, D. and the MHEEN group (2008) 'Is it worth investing in mental health promotion and prevention of mental illness? A systematic review of the evidence from economic evaluations'. *BMC Public Health* 8(20): 1471–2458.

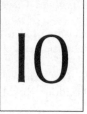

# 10

# Persistent and future challenges in public health

## *Susan R. Thompson*

## Climate change

In 2013 the Intergovernmental Panel on Climate Change (IPCC) confirmed that the world's climate is warming up, that the rate of this change is gathering momentum and that human influence was the dominant cause (IPCC 2013). The exception has been that in the last 15 years the average worldwide air temperature has remained stable, despite carbon dioxide emissions worldwide being at their highest level ever (IPCC 2013). Climate change is an extremely complex science and although more research is needed to formulate accurate projections it is anticipated that the world could be 2 degrees centigrade warmer by the end of the century. It is predicted that there will be more intense and frequent heatwaves, wet regions will receive more rainfall and dryer regions more and sustained periods of drought (IPCC 2013). In the UK the average temperature has risen by 0.25 degrees centigrade per decade since the 1960s, with summer rainfall decreasing and winter rainfall increasing (HPA 2012a). Heatwaves are felt most in urban areas and the last major heatwave in the UK in 2003 has been said to have caused an extra 2,000 deaths (Johnson *et al.* 2004). Researchers studying climate change and the probability of extreme weather conditions estimated that climate change had at least doubled the risk of such a heatwave occurring (Stott *et al.* 2004). Increased precipitation has also led to increased flooding both in the UK and globally (Pall *et al.* 2011). The dramatic levels of rainfall and flooding in the UK in the winter of 2013/14 made it the wettest on record and may be a consequence of global warming causing more intensive and heavier rainfall events (Met Office 2014). In addition to temperature and rainfall, reduced cloud cover increases exposure to harmful ultraviolet light, increasing the risks of developing skin cancer. Changes in humidity can worsen respiratory illnesses and increases the spread of infectious diseases (HPA 2012a). Although there is uncertainty around the effects of global warming, it is possible that melting polar ice will significantly lower the sea temperature, affecting the Gulf Stream, the warm surface water which gives the UK its mild winters. If this happens winter temperatures in the UK will fall by 5 degrees centigrade, resulting in winters more like those in Scandinavian countries. There is a concerted effort by climate change lobbyists to move conversations and actions on climate change more into the mainstream and disassociate climate change from its environmentalist/left-wing image and bring on board centre-right political parties around the world (COIN 2013). In this way cross-party support for measures to tackle climate change should be possible. Climate change will affect all of us to a greater or lesser extent, but those who will be mostly affected are those in developing countries and where subsistence is already marginal. Low-lying areas and small island states such as Bangladesh and the Pacific island of Myanmar are at significant risk of inundation due to rising sea levels. Extreme weather events such as drought or flooding impact on crop growth and cause soil erosion, which results in food insecurity and scarcity of clean water (UN General Assembly 2008). The health impact related to climate change is judged to be an increase in malnutrition, diarrhoeal disease, injury and death due to extreme weather conditions and a change in the distribution of some diseases such as malaria (UN General Assembly 2008). It is also thought that climate change may lead to mass migration and developed countries have expressed fear that they will be inundated with migrants fleeing unsustainable areas of the world (COIN 2013). Displacement causes its own health issues and is associated with vulnerability to disease, abuse and attack, and a myriad of psychological and physical health problems (UNHCR 2013). However, the evidence tends to suggest that the majority of migrants will resettle either temporarily or permanently within their own countries, most usually travelling from rural to urban areas (COIN 2013). Suggested solutions to limit the effect of climate change in vulnerable areas are: improved coastal protection, planting forests and mangroves to prevent inundation, the development of drought resistance crops, more irrigation systems and increased planning and provision of equipment to tackle emergencies when they arise; although funding to instigate such measures remains sparse (UN General Assembly 2008).

## Health protection

An important arm of public health work is protecting the public from harm caused by a variety of potential hazards. These include protection from radiation; chemical and environmental hazards; monitoring of infectious diseases; investigating the cause and responding to outbreaks of disease or international health alerts; and the testing of food, water or other environmental samples for pathogens harmful for health. In England these services are provided by the health protection department of Public Health England. Regional offices provide specialist support to health and local authorities, the emergency services and other relevant agencies regarding emergency planning for major events as well as microbiological testing for infectious disease. Health protection services also provide screening for new entrants to the UK and support to the immigration services, advising on the health status of potential migrants (Public Health England 2013a). Routine infectious disease work within the UK involves monitoring and responding to the regular outbreaks of norovirus, seasonal influenza and cryptosporidium infection. There are many health professionals whose prime role is that of health protection – environmental health officers who monitor, improve and enforce regulations relating to food safety, workplace health and safety, pollution levels and housing conditions, to give just some examples. Infection control nurses educate staff, patients and relatives regarding infection control measures in hospital and the home.

Pollution remains a serious health protection issue. There is undeniable evidence that air pollution contributes to disease. In 2006 The Committee on the Medical Effects of Air Pollution found that fine particles of pollutants breathed in on a daily basis were associated with increased CVD deaths (COMEAP 2006). Air pollution is also linked to the increased incidence and severity of asthma attacks; this in the UK despite the fact that clean air acts have made the air generally cleaner. It is thought that it is increased road traffic and vehicle emissions, especially from trucks, that have caused the increased levels of asthma (COMEAP 2010) and that those living within 500 metres of a busy road are more susceptible to pollution-related health problems (Health Effects Institute 2009).

## Sexual health

Sexually transmitted diseases (STIs) continue to rise in the UK, especially amongst young people and men who have sex with men. In 2012 there were half a million new infections, equating to a 5 per cent rise on the previous year. Chlamydia is the most common STI, and with the majority of sufferers experiencing no symptoms it is important especially for young people, who account for 64 per cent of all cases, to be tested regularly via the National Chlamydia Screening Programme. Genital warts and genital herpes are also increasing, with 54 per cent of cases in those under 25 years of age (Public Health England 2013b).

HIV remains a significant threat to the UK and the worldwide population. Great strides have been made in recent decades with the advent of anti-retro viral drugs; however, HIV infection causes significant loss of life and a reduced healthy life span. Treatment costs for HIV are high and strict compliance to regimes is necessary for treatment to be effective. However, these drugs are associated with side effects that can result in diminished quality of life. The provision of new drug therapy has led to increasing numbers of people living with the disease. In 2011 there were an estimated 96,000 people living with HIV in the UK, a quarter of whom were estimated to be untested and consequently unaware of their condition. Men in the UK are twice as likely as women to be HIV positive (HPA 2012b). The spread of HIV infection varies throughout the UK. In 2008 the number of people diagnosed as being HIV positive and living in London was almost 27,000. This compares dramatically with all other regions of the UK where rates are significantly lower, the lowest rate being just 1,000 in North-East England. Sources of infection were equally distributed between men who have sex with men and male–female sex (ONS 2012).

Increased microbial resistance is of importance in the fight against sexually transmitted diseases. In 2012 cases of gonorrhoea in the general population rose by 21 per cent and within the population of men who have sex with men by a staggering 37 per cent (Public Health England 2013b). The bacteria that causes gonorrhoea has developed resistance to a range of different treatments over the last few decades and has caused enough concern for a national programme to be set up in 2000 to monitor trends in susceptibility of the bacteria to current antimicrobial agents (Ison *et al.* 2013).

Increasing resistance to antibiotics makes it essential for health promoters to encourage safe sex and condom use, which will prevent STIs from being transmitted throughout populations.

## Liver disease

Liver disease has been increasing for many years within England and Wales and is now the fifth largest cause of death (ONS 2008). The three main types are alcoholic liver disease, non-alcoholic fatty liver disease (NAFLD) and hepatitis. NAFLD is related to obesity and is estimated to affect 20–30 per cent of the population of developed nations, the majority of which is undiagnosed (British Liver Trust 2013). Alcoholic liver disease is slow in onset and symptomless in the early stages, but persistent heavy drinking leads to an increase in fat within the liver and a decrease in function. Eventually scar tissue forms, causing cirrhosis. Cutting back on drinking allows the liver to repair itself and, dependent on the level of damage, the liver has excellent capacity to heal, but good nutrition is essential for this healing process. One of the barriers to seeking help is the stigma associated with being judged as being an alcoholic. However, the majority of people suffering from the effects of too much alcohol intake are not dependent drinkers, rather they regularly drink above the recommended level (British Liver Trust 2013). Health care professionals need to be more ready and proactive in the assessment of patients' level of alcohol consumption and provide brief advice and signposting to specialist services that are able to assess in more depth and discuss strategies for cutting down. Blood tests for liver function are also an important measure to gauge the existing level of damage. Dependent drinkers will require more specialist and probably longer-term support, possibly within substance misuse services, but the growing issue is excess 'social' drinking. There needs to be more services based in primary care, alongside other mainstream services such as quit smoking services, to remove the stigma associated with discussing excess alcohol intake. Staff with direct patient contact ought to be proficient in the use of alcohol assessment tools; merely embarrassingly asking clients 'how many units do you drink a week?' is insufficient. Answers depend on honesty, lack of self-consciousness and good knowledge of the unit system on the part of the client.

A well-recognised tool to assess alcohol intake in the general population is the Alcohol Use Disorders Identification Test (Babor *et al.* 2001). This is a flexible test, whose first three questions (out of a possible ten) have been shown to have an 86 per cent specificity (i.e. it identified those with a problem 86 per cent of the time).

Hepatitis is a viral infectious disease that affects liver function. Hepatitis A is usually a limiting acute condition; however, B and C are more serious and cause liver damage. They are transmitted through blood (and, in the case of hepatitis B, semen). A vaccination exists for hepatitis B and health professionals receive immunisation, but no vaccination is yet available for hepatitis C. Levels of hepatitis C continue to rise in the UK, with the latest report showing 215,000 cases with between a third and a half of all cases being related to injecting drug use (Public Health England 2013c). Once detected antiviral medication can effect a cure in many cases; however, due to the target population being a hard-to-reach group it poses challenges for both prevention and treatment for the disease. The aim is to prevent infections due to increasing awareness and adoption of preventative methods such as use of needle exchanges. More testing and diagnostics services need to be offered and there needs to be an increase in the uptake of treatment and care (Public Health England 2013c).

## Gambling

In 2005 the then Labour government in the UK relaxed the laws on gambling (UK Government 2005), making it more accessible than ever before in UK society, whether online, on television or face-to-face. It also became seemingly more socially acceptable, especially amongst young people, although research regarding this is still sparse. In 2012 the Commons Culture, Media and Sport Committee published a report looking into changes that had occurred as a result of the act. It concluded that 'gambling is now widely accepted in the UK as a legitimate entertainment activity', and the committee opted to 'support liberalisation of rules' (Commons Select Committee 2012). In the US, where gambling has historically been more prevalent than in the UK, with 29 per cent of adults estimated as having gambled in casinos within the last year, public health officials have started to examine the negative health effects associated with gambling. This is a response to a threefold increase in gambling during the last 40 years (Potenza *et al.* 2002).

Sustained gambling over a period of hours has been seen to greatly increase stress levels resulting in increased heart rate and cortisol levels and has been thought to cause cardiac arrest (Meyer *et al.* 2000). These are the short-term health effects; long-term dependence or pathological gambling obviously results in financial problems with the accompanying psychosocial ramifications of this both for the individual and their family. Problem gambling can cause family breakdown, domestic violence, criminal activity, loss and disruption to employment and social isolation. Money spent on gambling means less money for everyday essentials of life such as good housing, nutrition and payment of utility bills. It is estimated that for every individual who has a problem with gambling five to ten others in contact with that individual suffer the repercussions of the gambler's habit (AMA 2013). Gambling can become addictive, an addictive behaviour being defined as 'the continued engagement in a behaviour despite adverse consequences' (Potenza *et al.* 2002). Addictive gambling is closely linked to other addictive behaviours, with those with substance misuse problems seemingly to be more prone to gambling addiction (Cunningham-Williams *et al.* 1998). Pathological gambling is also associated with increased suicide risk, with one US study showing up to 24 per cent of pathological gamblers to have attempted suicide (DeCaria *et al.* 1996) and gambling cities such as Las Vegas having four times the number of completed suicides of the average US city (Philips *et al.* 1997). Are we in the UK fuelling a major health issue for the future? One of the most disturbing results of the act is the effect that it has had on deprived communities. Gambling disproportionately affects poorer communities, those communities desperate for a little extra cash and therefore tempted to risk a little to gain a lot (Wiseman 2006). It has also been found that those who gamble are more likely to smoke and drink to excess, and that those in ill health are three times more likely to be a problem gambler than those in good health (Griffiths *et al.* 2010). Local authorities are trying to limit the number of betting outlets, but are not proving successful. In 2013 Newham Council in London unsuccessfully fought to prevent another betting shop opening in its area (it already has a staggering 82 outlets, equating to six in every square mile) (*The Guardian* 2013). There is concern that such betting shops derive too much of their revenue from fixed-odds gaming machines rather than flexible-odds horse or dog racing. The 2005 legislation only allowed four such machines in any one shop, hence the proliferation of the number of shops to circumvent these restrictions. In January 2014 a Labour Party proposal to give local authorities powers to limit the numbers of gaming machines was defeated in the House of Commons. There appears to be a lack of any political will on the behalf of central government to restrict gambling which is a useful source of revenue, especially as offshore gaming companies are to be taxed at the same rate as domestic retailers.

Within the UK there is a lack of awareness of gambling as a health issue. Primary care practitioners are not trained in the assessment of clients regarding their gambling habits, despite there being a variety of assessment tools available. These are question-based and similar to alcohol screening questionnaires, asking whether clients have ever felt the need to lie about their gambling, experienced financial difficulties due to their gambling or felt that they had a problem controlling the amount and frequency of their gambling (Johnson *et al.* 1997; Sullivan 1999). Males and adolescents seem more at risk of gambling addiction than the rest of the population (Potenza *et al.* 1997).

Whilst acknowledging that problem gamblers existed, the government seems to think that this was best tackled by the gambling organisations themselves and by education, especially of young people (Commons Select Committee 2012). This is a common response to a health issue by governments, that of individual responsibility; that is, people are advised to resist temptation whilst the object of that temptation remains freely available.

# References

AMA (Australian Medical Association) (2013) *Health Effects of Problem Gambling*. Available online: https://ama.com.au/position-statement/health-effects-problem-gambling.

Babor, T.F., Higgins-Biddle, J.C., Saunders, J.B. and Monteiro, M.G. (2001) *The Alcohol Use Disorders Identification Test: Guidelines for use in primary care* (2nd edn). Copenhagen: Department of Mental Health and Substance Dependence, World Health Organization.

British Liver Trust (2013) *Alcohol*. Available online: http://79.170.44.126/britishlivertrust. org.uk/home-2/liver-information/liver-conditions/alcohol/.

COIN (Climate Outreach Information Network) (2013) *The Centre Right and Climate Change*. Available online: http://www.climateoutreach.org.uk/portfolio-item/a-new-conversation-with-the-centre-right-about-climate-change/.

COMEAP (The Committee on the Medical Effects of Air Pollutants) (2006) *Cardiovascular Disease and Air Pollution*. London: COMEAP.

COMEAP (The Committee on the Medical Effects of Air Pollutants) (2010) *Does Outdoor Air Pollution Cause Asthma?* London: COMEAP.

Commons Select Committee (2012) *The Gambling Act 2005: A bet worth taking?* London: Culture, Media and Sport Committee.

Cunningham-Williams, R.M., Cottler, L.B., Compton III, W.M. and Spitznagel, E.L. (1998) 'Taking chances: Problem gamblers and mental health disorders – results from the St. Louis Epidemiologic Catchment Area Study'. *American Journal of Public Health*: 1093–6.

DeCaria, C.M., Hollander, E., Grossman, R., Wong, C.M., Mosovich, S.A. and Cherkasky, S. (1996) 'Diagnosis, neurobiology, and treatment of pathological gambling'. *Journal of Clinical Psychiatry* (suppl 8): 80–3.

Griffiths, M., Wardle, H., Orford, J., Sproston, K. and Erens, B. (2010) 'Gambling, alcohol, consumption, cigarette smoking and health: Findings from the 2007 British Gambling Prevalence Survey'. *Addiction Research and Theory* 18(2): 208–32.

*The Guardian.* 'Newham Council Told to Accept Betting Shop It Rejected'. 17 June 2013.

The Health Effects Institute (2009) *Traffic-Related Air Pollution: A critical review of the literature on emissions, exposure, and health effects.* Boston, MA: HEI.

HPA (Health Protection Agency) (2012a) *Climate Change in the UK: Current evidence and projections.* London: HPA.

HPA (Health Protection Agency) (2012b) *HIV in the United Kingdom: 2012 Report.* London: HPA.

IPCC (Intergovernmental Panel on Climate Change) (2013) 'Human influence on climate clear'. Available online: http://www.ipcc.ch/news_and_events/docs/ar5/press_release_ar5_wgi_en.pdf.

Ison, C.A., Town, K., Obi, C., Chisholm, S., Hughes, G., Livermore, D.M. and Lowndes, C.M. (2013) 'Decreased susceptibility to cephalosporins among gonococci: Data from the Gonococcal Resistance to Antimicrobials Surveillance Programme (GRASP) in England and Wales, 2007–2011'. *Lancet Infectious Diseases* 13(9): 762–8.

Johnson, E.E., Hamer, R., Nora, R.M., Tan, B., Eisenstein, N. and Engelhart, C. (1997) 'The Lie/Bet screening tool for pathological gamblers'. *Psychological Report* 83(3, Pt 2): 1219–24.

Johnson, H., Kovats, S., McGregor, G., Stedman, J., Gibbs, M., Walton, H., and Cook, L. (2004) 'The impact of the 2003 heat wave on mortality and hospital admissions in England'. *Epidemiology* 15: 126.

The Met Office (2014) 'The recent storms and floods in the UK'. Available online: http://www.metoffice.gov.uk/media/pdf/1/2/Recent_Storms_Briefing_Final_SLR_20140211.pdf.

Meyer, G., Hauffa, B.P., Schedlowski, M., Pawluk, C., Stadler, M.A. and Exton, M.S. (2000) 'Casino gambling increases heart rate and salivary cortisol in regular gamblers'. *Biological Psychiatry* 48: 948–53.

ONS (Office for National Statistics) (2008) *Health Service Quarterly* 40(4): 59–60.

ONS (Office for National Statistics) (2012) *HIV Infection in England.* London: ONS.

Pall, P., Aina, T., Stone, D.A., Stott, P.A., Nozawa, T., Hilberts, A.G.J., Lohmann, D. and Allen, M.R. (2011) 'Anthropogenic greenhouse gas contribution to flood risk in England and Wales in autumn 2000'. *Nature* 470: 382–5.

Phillips, D.P., Welty, W.R. and Smith, M.M. (1997) 'Elevated suicide levels associated with legalized gambling'. *Suicide Life Threat Behaviour* 27: 373–8.

Potenza, M., Fiellin, D., Heninger, G., Rounsaville, B. and Mazure, C. (2002) 'An addictive behavior with health and primary care implications'. *Journal of General International Medicine* 17(9): 721–32.

Public Health England (2013a) http://www.hpa.org.uk/AboutTheHPA/.

Public Health England (2013b) *Sexually Transmitted Infections and Chlamydia Screening in England, 2012.* London: PHE.

Public Health England (2013c) *Hepatitis C in the UK: 2013 report.* London: PHE.

Stott, P.A., Stone, D.A. and Allen, M.R. (2004) 'Human contribution to the European heat-wave of 2003'. *Nature* 432: 610–14.

Sullivan, S. (1999) *Development of the 'EIGHT' Problem Gambling Screen.* PhD Thesis. Auckland, New Zealand: Auckland Medical School.

UK Government (2005) *Gambling Act 2005.*

UNHCR (United Nations High Commissioner for Refugees) (2013) Website: www.unhcr.org.

United Nations General Assembly (2008) *Climate Change and the Most Vulnerable Countries: The imperative to act.* Available online: http://www.un.org/ga/president/62/ThematicDebates/ccact/vulnbackgrounder1July.pdf.

Wiseman, J. (2006) 'State lotteries: Using state lotteries to fleece the poor'. *Journal of Economic Issues* 40(4): 955–66.

# Glossary

**Asylum seeker** – A person who has left their country of origin and lodged an application for asylum in another country and is waiting for the results of that application.

**Comparative needs** – Needs which arise from the requirement to ensure equity of provision to similar populations.

**Epidemiology** – The study of disease and health determinants within populations.

**Expressed needs** – Needs identified from the level of use of services already provided.

**Felt needs** – The health needs that are identified by people themselves.

**Health impact assessment** – Investigations into the possible negative wider ramifications of proposed interventions.

**Health literacy** – The level of knowledge of health issues and their determinants possessed by communities or individuals and their capacity to act on these.

**Incidence** – The number of new cases of a certain condition appearing in a population.

**Index of multiple deprivation (IMD)** – A measurement used to score the level of deprivation of local authority areas in the UK.

**Models** – Frameworks based on best practice that act as tools for health promoters to use to ensure effective working.

**Morbidity** – Suffering from a state of ill health, either physical or mental, as a result of a disease, illness or injury.

**Motivational interviewing (MI)**– A person-centred method of supporting individuals through behaviour change.

**Normative needs** – Health needs of a population decided upon by professionals as a result of studying epidemiological trends.

**Prevalence** – The number of cases of a certain condition present in a population at a certain time.

**Protected characteristics** – Nine characteristics identified by the UK Equality and Human Rights Commission which are liable to be the focus of discrimination and should therefore be protected. These are discrimination on the grounds of: age, gender, disability, sexual orientation, gender reassignment, civil partnerships, race, pregnancy and maternity, religion and belief.

**Refugee** – According to the 1951 UN Convention on Refugees, someone 'owing to a well-founded fear of being persecuted for reasons of race, religion, nationality, membership of a particular social group, or political opinion, is outside the country of his nationality, and is unable to or, owing to such fear, is unwilling to avail himself of the protection of that country or who, not having a nationality and being outside the country of his former habitual residence as a result of such events, is unable or, owing to such fear, is unwilling to return to it'. Those granted refugee status have a right to remain in the country granting it.

**Self-efficacy** – An individual's belief that they will have the motivation and ability to undertake successful behavior change.

**Sensitivity (of screening test)** – The level of which the test is able to detect all those with the disease or trait that test is designed to detect.

**Specificity (of screening test)** – The level of which the test accurately detects only those with the disease or trait being screened for.

**Social epidemiology** – The study of the social factors that influence health.

**Social gradient of health** – Term describing that the lower a person's level is in society, the worse their health.

**Social marketing** – The use of advertising industry techniques to persuade individuals to change their attitudes and behaviour.

**Stakeholders** – Agencies, organisations and client groups with a connection to a particular health issue or community.

**Standardised mortality ratio (SMR)** – The SMR is used to compare the mortality risk of a study population to that of a standard population. The standard population is stated as 100, therefore a figure of under 100 for a specific population suggests fewer than expected deaths, whereas a figure of over 100 indicates more than expected deaths. SMR is often used to compare different geographical areas and population groups.

# Index